Disabling Diseases

*Physical, environmental and psychosocial
management*

Edited by

Andrew Frank

*Consultant Physician in Rheumatology and Rehabilitation, Northwick Park Hospital,
Harrow*

Peter Maguire

Senior Lecturer in Psychiatry, University of Manchester

Heinemann Medical Books

To our wives
Cynthia and Maggie
for their forbearance
and support

Heinemann Medical Books
An imprint of Heinemann Professional Publishing
Halley Court, Jordan Hill, Oxford OX2 8EJ

OXFORD   LONDON   MELBOURNE   AUCKLAND

First published 1988

British Library Cataloguing in Publication Data
Frank, Andrew O.
  Disabling diseases: physical,
  environmental and psychological
  management
  1. Sick persons. Care
  I. Frank, Andrew O.   II. Maguire, Peter
  362.1
ISBN 0-433-00057-0

Filmset by Eta Services (Typesetters) Ltd, Beccles, Suffolk
Printed in Great Britain by Redwood Burn Ltd, Trowbridge

Contents

iv *Contents*

Contributors

A. O. Frank, Consultant in Rheumatology and Rehabilitation, Northwick Park Hospital, Watford Road, Harrow HA1 3UJ.

G. P. Maguire, Senior Lecturer in Psychiatry, The University Hospital of South Manchester, West Didsbury, Manchester M20 8LR.

Nan Brady, Nurse Teacher, Salford School of Nursing, Peel House, Eccles, Manchester M30 0NJ.

M. Brill, Formerly Principal Officer of Policy and Planning, Social Services Department, Civic Centre, Harrow HA1 2UL.

A. J. Burnfield, Consultant in Child and Family Psychiatry, The Family Consultancy, Andover Health Centre, Charlton Road, Andover, Hampshire SP10 3JL.

Miss E. S. Glossop, Retired District Physiotherapist, Field House, Hawkswick, Skipton, North Yorkshire BD23 5QA.

Miss F. Hasler, Director of Islington Disablement Association, 90–92 Upper Street, London N1 0NP.

Miss J. Hills, Superintendent Physiotherapist, Northwick Park Hospital, Watford Road, Harrow HA1 3UJ.

M. Hodkinson, Professor of Geriatric Medicine, University College Hospital, London WC1E 6AU.

Mrs S. Homewood, Manager, Bentley Day Centre, 94 Uxbridge Road, Harrow Weald HA7 4LP.

D. J. Lane, Consultant Physician, Churchill Hospital, Headington, Oxford OX3 7LJ.

P. Morris-Jones, Reader in Paediatric Oncology, Royal Manchester Childrens Hospital, Pendlebury, Manchester M27 1HA.

Mrs C. Norton, Formerly Continence Adviser, Disabled Living Foundation, 380 Harrow Road, London W9 2BU.

M. Oliver, Principal Lecturer in Special Needs, Thames Polytechnic, Avery Hill Campus, Bexley Road, London SE9 2PQ.

R. A. Sellwood, Professor of Surgery, Withington Hospital, West Didsbury, Manchester M20 8LR.

Miss E. Yates, District Occupational Therapist, Northwick Park Hospital, Watford Road, Harrow HA1 3UJ.

Acknowledgements

We are indebted to many colleagues within Harrow Health District and Harrow Social Services for assistance in the production of this book. We are particularly grateful to Miss A. Shields for her assistance with the illustrations, and to Mrs M. Murphy and Mrs J. Watson for their invaluable secretarial assistance.

We are also indebted to Miss J. Bragg, Mr K. DeWitt, Dr A. J. M. Frank, Mr G. Harris, Mrs G. Hethershaw, Mrs J. Hughes, Miss S. MacDonald, Sister McRoberts, Miss M. Meikle, Dr N. Mitchell, Mr B. Mullan, Mr J. Norris, Mrs M. Richards, Mrs K. Ross-Smith, Mrs J. Sayers, Mr C. Sherratt, Miss R. Trevan, Miss J. Wade, Prof. M. Warren, Mr N. Webb and Mrs R. Whitcomb, for their help and expertise which they have made freely available. In particular we would like to thank Dr E. B. Raftery who kindly reviewed the chapter on coronary rehabilitation; his comments added greatly to the chapter.

We are indebted to Souvenir Press for permission to reproduce Figures 8.2 and 8.3 from *Multiple Sclerosis: A Personal Exploration*, by Alexander Burnfield; to Mr N. Wells for permission to reproduce Figure 2.1 from *Back Pain* (Office of Health and Economics, 1985), and to Margaret Holbrook for permission to reproduce Figure 5.2 from the *Journal of the Royal College of Physicians of London*. We are also indebted to Graham Hulme for permission to reproduce Figure 5.4 which was first shown in Bentley Day Centre Photography Exhibition in 1987.

Finally, we are grateful to Richard Barling of Heinemann Medical Books for his help throughout the preparation of this book.

Introduction

Medical education, at both undergraduate and postgraduate levels, is primarily based on the philosophy that by understanding the underlying nature of a disease process, treatment may be given with a view to obtaining a cure. This model of medical practice is perfectly satisfactory for a person who develops pneumonia or has a hernia which can be treated directly by medical or surgical means. It is, however, totally inappropriate for a large number of conditions which result in varying degrees of disability.

Within the caring professions there is a vast pool of expertise that can improve the quality of life for patients suffering from incurable disease or disability. Consequently the editors have joined with colleagues from the caring professions to look at different conditions from various perspectives. The end result is nearly always to demonstrate the devastating effect that these conditions can have on individuals, their families and friends.

All diseases are potentially disabling, either physically or mentally, and the disabling effects may be ameliorated in full or in part by skilled care. Two groups of diseases may result in severe dependence on others at great cost to personal, family and community resources. The largest group is that of locomotor disability largely caused by arthritis. Since few people actually die from arthritic disorders, the prevalence rises to an estimated 860 severely handicapped people within a population of 250 000.

Conversely, neurological disorders, although much less frequent (stroke 340, multiple sclerosis 80 in a similar population) may have more devastating social consequences. After a stroke a pattern of recovery can be expected when both physical and social rehabilitation are vital. This is explained in detail in Chapter 5. A similar rehabilitation process is required after accident or injury, which may be particularly complicated after a head injury when loss of intellectual function and personality changes create great difficulty for staff, family and friends.

Where the illness may deteriorate over time, as in most dementias or progressive neurological disorders such as multiple strokes, motor neurone disease or muscular dystrophy, psychological and physical support for patient and family need to be carefully planned and provided as required to meet the needs of the individual. Thus severe disability in a context of possible deterioration is described in detail in Chapter 8, on multiple sclerosis. Only rarely should it be impossible to support people in the community if adequate physical and emotional support are provided to both patient and carers by health and social services in close collaboration. Such support, however, may be very costly. Parkinson's disease is not discussed, in view of its good response to sophisticated medical management in many cases, although those suffering from this disease may need physiotherapy and physical support in the home, as well as support for their carers.

Finally, some diseases have an expectation of death. In some the critical phase may pass (cardiopulmonary problems in particular – see Chapters 3 and 4) but with cancer the fear of progression to death is always very real and thus three chapters (9–11) discuss the difficulties of helping people with some specific forms of cancer. In these chapters the need for clear honest communication between patient, family and professionals is explored in some depth.

In most disorders discussed, except for spinal pain or cardiopulmonary disease, there is the risk of possible disfigurement with all the additional psychological problems involved. The fear of disfigurement by disease (Chapter 1), or surgery (Chapters 10 and 11) may be more disabling than actually living with the loss of self-image and confidence that usually follows disfigurement. This is therefore discussed in some detail in the chapters on arthritis and cancer.

Disabilities may arise from accidents or illnesses for which a partial or total recovery is expected. Examples are the simple episode of back pain (Chapter 2), a coronary (Chapter 4) or stroke (Chapter 5). Here, after the initial shock, expectations of improvement aid adjustment. Other conditions may have an uncertain course, such as rheumatoid arthritis (Chapter 1), or multiple sclerosis (Chapter 8) and helping people adjust to uncertainty is a major problem in itself for patients and carers alike. Finally, some conditions are likely to progress relentlessly and here adjustment to increasing disability and the likelihood of dying require further help (Chapter 10).

The importance of the physical environment is stressed particularly in Chapters 1 and 5 on arthritis and stroke. As physical disability restricts mobility, the nature of the environment becomes very important. Thus those factors which influence the site of the home, adaptation of the dwelling (e.g. to facilitate living from a wheelchair or the relationship of the staircase to the site of the toilet) and the importance of equipment (aids) in the preservation of personal independence are all explored.

The first two chapters, on arthritis and spinal pain, have a strong bias towards physical methods of treatment with an emphasis on the role chartered physiotherapists can play in alleviating the effects of arthritis. Chapter 3 on disabling breathlessness emphasizes how a thorough understanding of pulmonary physiology can help in the management of this common problem. It is hoped that in time our understanding of disease will enable rehabilitation to be placed on a more scientific basis, as is demonstrated in this chapter. Helping people after a heart attack (Chapter 4) or stroke (Chapter 5) involves an understanding of the emotional changes consequent to the onset of a sudden life-threatening condition; the emphasis in these chapters is on assisting individuals in regaining their self-confidence and independence and their families in adjusting to a very changed situation. As the majority of disabled people are in the older age group, two chapters illustrate common problems. The first problem, incontinence (Chapter 6), may have devastating effects, but the provision of appropriate expertise within the community can transform the plight of many of those affected. The chapter on multiple disabilities (Chapter 7) is written by a consultant geriatrician because this is predominantly, although not exclusively, a problem of old age.

Chapters 8–11 review the effects that multiple sclerosis, leukaemia in childhood, carcinoma of the breast and a colostomy have on families, with a major emphasis on how patients can be helped to come to terms with the uncertainties associated with progressive illnesses giving rise to possible disability or death.

Chapter 12 outlines the importance of self-help and demonstrates the effective way in which people with spinal injuries support themselves through a dynamic group. The penultimate chapter (13) outlines the resources available from social services departments, which are often underutilized. The final chapter illustrates the vast range of help available to disabled people through both the voluntary sector and government departments.

Throughout the book the emphasis is on the physical, environmental and psychological aspects of care, placed in the context of contemporary medical practice where necessary.

It is hoped that this book makes clear the real desire on the part of the caring professions for people disabled through illness or injury to continue to take responsibility for their lives and to refute the idea that the professionals always wish to take charge. We firmly believe that the caring professions have a responsibility to help their clients understand the nature of their problems, the likely effects on the whole family and to aid adjustment so that the best decisions are made in the light of this knowledge.

Whilst the stimulus for this book has come from the awareness of the inadequacies of medical education in the field of disabling conditions, we recognize the almost total lack of multidisciplinary postgraduate training in this area, and that only close collaboration can succeed in providing the best opportunity for individuals to lead fulfilled lives in spite of disability.

It is hoped that this book will be of interest not only to doctors, in hospital or in the community, but also to members of the nursing, remedial, and social work professions.

A. Frank
Consultant Physician
Department of Rehabilitation
Northwick Park Hospital

P. Maguire
Senior Lecturer
Department of Psychiatry
University of Manchester

1

Arthritis

Andrew Frank and Sonia Glossop

INTRODUCTION AND EPIDEMIOLOGY

Arthritic conditions are the commonest disabling diseases, and thus warrant early consideration in this book. It is likely that there are approximately 860 people in each health district of 250 000 people who are severely, or very severely, disabled with some form of arthritis. The prevalence is even more staggering, with estimates of between 32 000–72 500 people with osteoarthritis in the average health district, and up to 6000 people with rheumatoid arthritis.[1] Each group practice of 10 000 patients might have up to 2900 people with osteoarthritis, and up to 250 people suffering from rheumatoid arthritis. Whilst the prevalence of osteoarthritis increases with age, it is not always appreciated that arthritis afflicts people of all ages, including children.

Where possible, it is the job of the doctor to modify the course of the disease. Where this is not possible, the maximum symptomatic help should be given. Whilst doctors are well informed about the various drug therapies, they are not always so well informed about alternative ways in which people can be helped. This chapter discusses in some detail physical methods of treatment, particularly as given by chartered physiotherapists, and also environmental, psychological and social aspects of management. It is not proposed to examine the usual treatment of any form of arthritis, as these aspects are well covered in the standard texts.

PATTERNS OF ARTHRITIS

Childhood arthritis

Arthritis may rarely present in children; in these cases the umbrella term of 'juvenile chronic arthritis' is used. It may present as an acute illness – Still's disease – and in the course of time, features characteristic of adult inflammatory polyarthropathy may develop, often as ankylosing spondylitis or rheumatoid arthritis. Many general practitioners will not see this condition. As with all childhood conditions, time spent explaining the nature of the condition to parents, and active encouragement to support their children's attempts to maintain as near a normal childhood as possible, both at school and at leisure, are critical. The disease may be disabling, with increased risk of infections, iridocyclitis leading to visual impairment and severe disabilities in adult life. [2]

Adult inflammatory arthritis

The causes of arthritis are not clearly understood. The two major groups are the inflammatory arthritides and osteoarthritis, or 'degenerative' arthritis. Within the former group, rheumatoid arthritis predominates, with an estimated prevalence of between 100–250 per 10 000 population. [1] Its diagnostic and clinical features are documented elsewhere.

It must be noted that a positive test for rheumatoid factor by itself does not confirm the diagnosis, as this may be present in other conditions, and in the normal population. Poor control with regular non-steroidal anti-inflammatory drugs (NSAIDs), the presence of high rheumatoid factor titres, systemic illness, nodules or vasculitis should suggest that the disease is likely to take a progressive course which warrants a specialist opinion.

It is not the purpose of this chapter to outline details of management, but general practitioners will wish to attempt to control pain and stiffness with NSAIDs (see pp. 13–15, 48–9), with additional analgesics regularly or as required. The role of local steroid injections is generally agreed to be valuable for flares of disease activity in certain joints, and should not be given more frequently than 3-monthly in any joint. The prudently timed injection may give immeasurable relief for important occasions such as weddings or holidays.

Other inflammatory arthritides

Other forms of disabling inflammatory arthritis include the spondylarthritides which include ankylosing spondylitis, Reiter's syndrome, the arthritis of ulcerative colitis or Crohn's disease, and psoriasis. It is important to distinguish this group of disorders, not only as the spinal deformity can be prevented in many instances, but also because of the medical implications. There is a genetic predisposition, usually linked to the B27 genotype, to the other spondylarthritides. A similar, though smaller, predisposition exists for other family members.

The less common polyarthropathy following viral infections is often self-limiting. The special features of infectious arthritis (including gonorrhoea), reactive arthritis and other miscellaneous arthropathies (e.g. sarcoidosis) are outside the province of this chapter, and will often require specialist advice.

Gout has certain important features. It is often misdiagnosed on the basis of hyperuricaemia, and most rheumatologists require the aspiration of urate crystals from a joint to confirm the diagnosis. The presence of hyperuricaemia may alert the physician to the presence of hypertension or hyperlipidaemia which may require treatment. Gout induced in older people by diuretics can often be prevented by adjustment of therapy for the underlying disorder so that the need for diuretics is decreased. Recurrent attacks of gout can usually be prevented by the use of allopurinol, started after resolution of an acute attack, and with initial cover with appropriate NSAIDs.

Ankylosing spondylitis

It is important to diagnose ankylosing spondylitis as it is believed that proper supervision can prevent deformities. It classically presents as low back pain in young people, usually men, and is often diagnosed by the detection of sacroiliitis radiologically. It is familial with an increased incidence of other spondylarthritides (see above). Rarely the disease affects the spine and spares the sacroiliac joints. Not infrequently an inflammatory peripheral arthritis is noted, usually affecting the large joints.

It is believed that there is a focal inflammatory process at the site of ligamental attachments, which may subsequently give rise to calcification and ossification. The pain and morning stiffness is more pronounced than in mechanical back pain, may be associated with an elevated erythrocyte sedimentation rate, and is often eased by the longer-acting NSAIDs or exercise. Phenylbutazone may be prescribed for this condition by consultant rheumatologists as it is often more effective than other non-steroidal drugs, for reasons that are not clear.

It is important to confirm or exclude the diagnosis for any particular individual. When growth has stopped, scanning the sacroiliac joints may be helpful if x-rays are normal and the genetic predisposition may be confirmed by the finding of the B27 genotype. The presence of the B27 genotype does not of itself confirm the diagnosis.

As in all disabling or potentially disabling conditions, the social assessment (pp. 6–7) is important, particularly in noting the effects of the disease on employment and leisure. It is rare for this condition to be severely disabling. When it is, these effects can be ameliorated in part by the means explored later in this chapter.

Management of ankylosing spondylitis

Physiotherapy is the key to management. Failure to attend for therapy or reassessment is often a problem as pain is not always a dominant symptom, and stiffness not always a noticeable disability at the beginning. General practitioners must emphasize the importance of physiotherapy to their patients with this condition.

The *physical assessment* should be recorded using charts so that objective measurements are available on reassessment. Movements of the cervical spine can be measured with a goniometer, and the anterior Schoeber's test used to measure lumbar spine movement. Spinal and hip flexion is measured by the 'fingertip-to-floor' measurement; flexion deformity of the neck by the 'tragus-of-the-ear-to-the-wall' distance; chest expansion is measured to detect costovertebral joint involvement; and the height of the patient is recorded. Using objective parameters, the patient can see the changes in mobility consequent to the performance of exercises and the loss of mobility consequent to neglecting exercises.

For *postural management*, patients are advised to sleep on a firm mattress using one or no pillows, and to sit in a firm high-backed armchair which supports the neck. Patients are encouraged to lie prone, either on the bed before going to sleep, or on the floor to watch the television in the evening. Patients with a fixed kyphosis, or loss of hip extension, are encouraged to lie supine, adjusting pillows or using foam rubber to support the spine.

The objectives of *physiotherapy* are listed in Table 1.1. It is important that patients understand why the exercises are recommended, and see this as a

Table 1.1 Objectives of physiotherapy in ankylosing spondylitis

Prevent stiffness and deformity through exercises

Maintain range of movement of spinal joints

Maintain range of movement of peripheral joints

Maintain range of movement of costovertebral joints

Maintain an upright posture

Maintain general physical fitness to augment points 1–5 above

Educate the patient about the disease to encourage intelligent compliance with advice

If desired, encourage membership of the National Ankylosing Spondylitis Society vital part of living with the disease. Many patients find that their stiffness is markedly reduced if regular exercises are performed.

Patients need to continue in their regular employment and should be given appointment times to fit in with their work, which often means providing an evening appointment if necessary.

Following the initial assessment, the patient's needs are met either by individual treatment, or by attending a group exercise programme. This programme must include exercises for extension, flexion and rotation of the cervical, thoracic and lumbar spines. Hip extension exercises are also included. Breathing exercises are of prime importance and should be taught to relate to any body position in lying, sitting and standing, thus encouraging the patient to practise deep breathing frequently throughout the day.

If other joints are involved, exercises specifically relating to these joints, for instance shoulders, hips, knees and ankles, are taught.

The provision of an illustrated booklet will remind and encourage the patient to do exercises at home. Booklets are available from the National Ankylosing Spondylitis Society (see Chapter 14), which also produces an accompanying cassette. As well as illustrated exercises, the booklet provides much useful information about the disease and its treatment. A similar booklet is produced by the Arthritis and Rheumatism Council (Appendix 1.1).

Hydrotherapy is important in the treatment of ankylosing spondylitis, as the warmth of the water usually relieves muscle spasm and pain and water allows for greater freedom of movement. Exercises taught in the pool can be carried out by the patient in his or her local swimming baths and regular visits to the baths must be encouraged. Patients who have problems in attending regularly for treatment because of employment difficulties should be offered the opportunity of attending for a 1-week intensive course of exercises and hydrotherapy.

Physical fitness is of prime importance and activities such as swimming, badminton and running should be encouraged, as they will increase the breathing capacity. Circuit work in the gymnasium as part of a group activity programme should include rowing, cycling, sit-ups and press-ups. Discussion time and counselling during a group session will provide support and improve the patient's motivation, which is often difficult to maintain.

Reassessment of mobility should coincide with an outpatient clinic appointment so that any deterioration in mobility, or problems which need discussing, can be reported to the medical staff. A further course of physiotherapy may be recommended where loss of mobility has been demonstrated.

A patient may be referred in the late stage of the disease following default, or when the disease has not been diagnosed and treated in the early stages. It is important to treat the patient actively and intensively in order to obtain and maintain any increase in mobility that is still possible.

Osteoarthritis (OA)

This is an extremely common group of conditions, the causes of which remain unclear. Approximately one-fifth of all people on a general practitioner's list will have OA.[1] Doctors frequently refer to OA as 'wear and tear' arthritis, and this is useful as patients can realize that it is distinct from the inflammatory arthritides which are usually more aggressive. Whilst mechanical factors undoubtedly play a part in aetiology, other factors are important. Certain forms run in families. The prevalence of OA increases with age, contributing to the multiple handicaps which may limit independence in old age.

The medical management of OA is similar to that of inflammatory arthritis in the use of analgesics, NSAIDs and the local injection of steroids. No second-line drugs have been shown to be helpful. We believe, however, that much more can be done to help people with arthritis than drug management alone, and the main objective of this chapter is to outline these measures in more detail.

ASSESSMENT OF ARTHRITIS

Social assessment

Young doctors may still be taught at medical school that a social history consists of a knowledge of smoking and drinking habits. For those with arthritis, the following information is important, but the principles of the social history are the same as for many disabling conditions.

The details of accommodation are important. Inside the house, are there stairs? People with disabling conditions which are likely to deteriorate are helped if they live in a ground-floor flat, or a bungalow. If they live in a house, could they become independent on the ground floor? Can they manage the steps outside the house?

The site of the toilet may be critical, particularly in old age when urgency and frequency may be a problem. Is the downstairs toilet inside? Does the patient shower, or struggle in and out of a bath? Are there difficulties with dressing? Are there any other difficulties with daily living tasks?

What support is given by the family, either the spouse, or relatives living elsewhere? Do they help practically with the housework, cooking or shopping? Do any friends and neighbours fill this role? The understanding of the family is also critical as they may have a great influence on the patient. Some families are supportive and understanding. Some may be too supportive, and need counselling as to how much or how little help they should give.

People with arthritis have other concerns apart from the basic problems of independent living. There may be difficulties at work, or getting to work. Driving may be difficult. Hobbies may be more important for some people than work or housework, and for a few may be the main motivating factor.

These areas will be influenced in different ways by arthritis. Restrictions in activity may be due to an acute exacerbation in one or more joints, and resolve as the exacerbation settles. Conversely, for those unfortunate enough to suffer from severe deforming arthritis, these difficulties may become progressive. Not all doctors will feel able to look into every area, but it is important that an experienced person who understands the effects of arthritis on patients and their families does this. It may be a member of the primary health care team or the hospital team. Physiotherapists who advise patients in the physical aspects of self-care may be well qualified to explore these areas with patients, and indeed cannot advise regarding physical management without an awareness of the social situation.

Physical assessment of peripheral arthropathy

In the same way that physicians monitor disease activity regularly, the effect of any arthropathy on individual joints needs to be documented, together with the subsequent disability. Such monitoring is often neglected by physicians, but may be performed by another member of the rheumatology team, e.g. physiotherapists. A joint range chart will indicate the joints affected by stiffness, and by how much. A chart of the patient's ability to carry out daily living activities should be kept, with notes taken of where help is required. A checklist is provided in Table 1.2. The physical assessment provides guidelines on which to base treatment, and may detect patients who need advice on joint protection, or who should be seen by an occupational therapist (see below).

MANAGEMENT OF ARTHRITIS

Physical

Aims for physiotherapy in inflammatory arthritis
The objectives are outlined in Table 1.3. The chartered physiotherapist

Table 1.2   Checklist for people with arthritis

---

1 Can you get easily
    in and out of bed?
    on and off the toilet?
    in and out of your armchair?
    in and out of the bath?
2 Do you need help with
    washing/bathing?
    dressing?
    eating?
3 Can you manage steps and stairs?
4 How far can you walk?
5 What prevents you from walking further?
6 Are your shoes comfortable?
7 Has your arthritis affected your work/housework, or your ability to get to work?
8 Can you use all the kitchen utensils?
9 How does arthritis affect your marital (and/or sexual) relationship?
10 Has your arthritis caused you to feel particularly miserable, low, tense or 'on edge'?
11 Are there any other personal or practical problems about which you wish to ask?

---

must try to maintain the patient's mobility or to improve it where function has been lost. It is essential to try to prevent deformity as a flexion contracture is difficult to treat once it has occurred.

Where there is pain and joint stiffness, muscles become weak and contractures can occur. Muscle strength and tone must therefore be maintained. Relief of pain and muscle spasm should be considered as part of treatment though not in isolation. In the past, time was spent on using physiotherapy as a placebo with the use of various forms of heat for pain relief without

Table 1.3   Objectives of physiotherapy in peripheral arthropathy

---

Relief of pain and muscle spasm to facilitate:

Maintenance of muscle strength and tone

Improve or maintain range of joint movement to prevent deformity and contractures

Improve functional activities, i.e. walking

Advise patients about the effects of activity on their joints and to learn 'joint protection'

Teach a programme of home exercises to meet individual needs

Assessment for pain control using physical methods e.g. transcutaneous electrical nerve stimulation (TENS) or acupuncture (Fig. 1.1)

---

following this up with exercises to improve mobility. The patient must learn how to maintain his or her own joint mobility physically at home. Some physical measures for the management of chronic pain (e.g. transcutaneous electrical nerve stimulation; Fig. 1.1) are discussed in Chapter 2.

Methods of treatment

Treatment may involve teaching the patient a programme of home exercises, supplying him or her with an illustrated exercise booklet and reviewing progress at regular intervals, fixed to coincide with clinic appointments.

A number of individual treatment sessions may be arranged when the patient is in need of a supervised programme. Various forms of heat may be used, which can include wax baths, hot packs, or short-wave diathermy, prior to exercises being given. Ice packs used on a warm or swollen joint give relief to some patients; the chartered physiotherapist must first make sure that the condition of the patient's skin is satisfactory. Oil should be used on trophic skin first. Active rather than passive exercises must be given; the exercises may be resisted by adding weights and springs or manual resistance to increase muscle strength. Hydrotherapy is one of the most useful forms of treatment, since exercises are made easier by the buoyancy of the water with loss of friction. The temperature of the water is kept at approximately 97 C as the warmth helps to relieve muscle spasm, allowing for an increase in the range of joint movement. Children with juvenile chronic arthritis respond particularly well to hydrotherapy and enjoy the freedom which the water gives them. A hydrotherapy treatment session must always be followed up with 'dry land' exercises, and home exercises taught.

Frequent and regular review of patients who do home exercises encourages them to follow their programme as the physiotherapist will know when they have not been doing so!

Patients at work appreciate a physiotherapy review date which coincides with their outpatient clinic appointment, where an up-to-date report can be made to the doctor and splints (p. 11) reviewed. The patient has the opportunity to discuss any new problems or worries. Where deterioration in the patient's affected joints are noted at the review, a course of physiotherapy can be given to try and improve the situation. Patients should not be given long-standing physiotherapy without review. Treatment given when needed is more effective.

Elderly patients and those with severe disabling disease are not always helped by hospital physiotherapy. The difficulties created for the patient by irregular and time-consuming ambulance journeys do not help. The journey may be long, the ride rough, and sitting waiting for the transport either

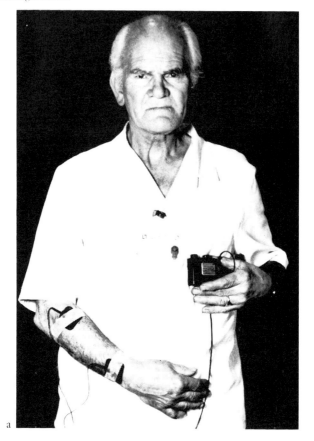

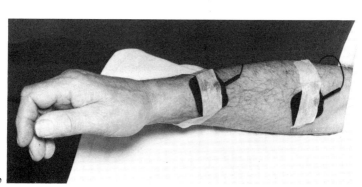

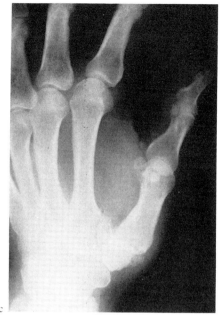

c

Fig. 1.1a–c Intractable pain from osteoarthritis of the carpometacarpal joint of the thumb unresponsive to medication or injection. Response to transcutaneous electrical nerve stimulation facilitates continuation in employment. The stimulator rests easily within the breast-pocket of the patient's tunic

before or after treatment does not encourage mobility. Domiciliary physiotherapy (Fig. 1.2) should be provided for this category of patient, giving the therapist a more realistic view of the patient's problems at home; the physiotherapist can then take the opportunity of giving relatives and community nurses advice on the physical management of the patient.

Splinting

Splints may be used to prevent or decrease deformity, and also to protect joints from stress and strain whilst the patient is working, doing household jobs or gardening. They may be made of a variety of materials, using different forms of plastic. Serial splints, usually made from plaster of Paris or of plastic which is easily remoulded when heated, are used to decrease a joint deformity gradually. By stretching the tight structures around a joint with exercise and stretching, particularly following hydrotherapy, a new plaster or remoulded plastic splint can be applied at regular intervals until a more satisfactory joint position has been obtained.

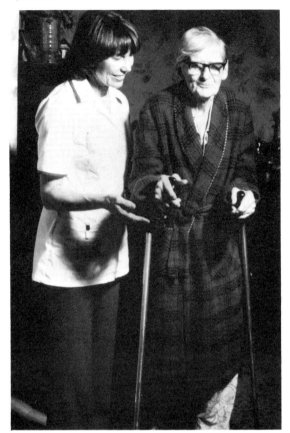

Fig. 1.2   Use of domiciliary physiotherapy to maximize mobility within the home

Resting splints should be provided for patients where deformity is increasing but is correctable. This applies particularly to patients developing ulnar drift at the metacarpophalangeal joints. The splints should be worn at night wearing one on each hand on alternate nights. Trying to wear both at once often results in inability to turn over in bed.

Ready-made working splints are obtainable and these may be suitable for some patients, particularly if the wrist joints are painful. Other patients require their splints to be individually moulded and these should be provided by the orthotist or therapist.

'Lively' splints may be provided following reconstructive hand surgery, particularly involving tendon repair where the patient is able to exercise his or her fingers within a limited range to maintain joint mobility and muscle strength.

Once splints are provided the patient should be seen at regular intervals to ensure that they fit correctly and do not require adjustment or replacing. An uncomfortable splint does not do the job for which it has been made, nor is it worn.

Joint protection

This important subject needs to be discussed with patients whatever the stage of their disease, as they will often unknowingly traumatize a joint through trying to maintain their independence.

A chair which is too low and therefore difficult to get out of will increase the strain on knees and also on the hands, wrists and elbows in the struggle to get up. Sticks and crutches will help to relieve the strain on painful hips and knees, though these should be chosen carefully as the grip of the stick and crutch can again put unnecessary strain on the hands and wrists, and when needed a 'rubberzote' hand grip can be added, or forearm (trough) crutches supplied instead.

The height of the crutches and sticks requires individual measurement. If too high or too low, walking aids will add to the patient's postural and joint problems by causing increased pressure on the joints of the upper limbs or by forcing the patients into a stooping posture.

Working wrist splints may be worn to prevent trauma to the wrists for many jobs, including housework. Patients should be advised on simple ideas in the home, such as half-filling a pan or kettle, adding more water separately if required; sliding pans across an even surface from the cooker and not lifting heavy objects; keeping groceries and dishes on a lower shelf instead of struggling to reach up; using long-handled sweeping brushes to avoid having to kneel down; having a shower to prevent struggling in and out of a bath; a duvet for ease in bed-making, and clothes with a front fastening to relieve the struggle if shoulders are painful (see pp. 24–7). Many other useful tips may be found from reading self-help leaflets published by the Arthritis and Rheumatism Council (see Appendix 1.1).

Drug management

The aims of drug therapy in arthritis are listed in Table 1.4. Morning stiffness may be very severe, and slows the process of getting up and about, particularly in rheumatoid arthritis, but also in osteoarthritis. Although drug therapy is detailed in the standard texts, the following points are not given

Table 1.4 Aims of drug management in arthritis

Modify the underlying disease process
Reduce joint inflammation
Decrease morning stiffness
Minimize pain from inflamed or damaged joints
Maintain function by prophylactic analgesia
Minimize side-effects of treatment, e.g. dyspepsia
Treat complications of disease or disability, e.g. depression

enough emphasis. There has been a tendency in recent years to commence disease-modifying drugs in rheumatoid arthritis much earlier, sometimes within weeks or months of the onset of the disease. When patients are not settling quickly after regular NSAIDs, a specialist opinion should be obtained with a view to starting treatment with disease-modifying drugs. A short discussion on the role of NSAIDs appears on pp. 48–9. It is particularly important to use the long-acting NSAIDs at night in order to minimize the distress of getting up in the morning.

The role of analgesia is most critical and is not given the attention it deserves. Many patients taking NSAIDs do not realize that they may take analgesics in addition. During acute exacerbations of the disease, analgesics may be required regularly, but more usually they are taken as needed. Three points are worth stressing. Firstly, all too often patients are given only mild analgesics (paracetamol or the paracetamol-containing compounds), even when it is clear that they are ineffective. This is demoralizing, and unnecessarily exposes the patient to the risks of side-effects. Particularly for the younger patient, who is less likely to have side-effects from the more potent analgesics, the stronger analgesics such as buprenorphine, nefopam, or meptazinol should be considered.

The second point is that it is extremely important in the battle to preserve morale, and to minimize the risks of depression, that patients know that if they are really at 'rock bottom' and in severe pain, they have available to them a drug that is effective. Even patients who are reluctant to take tablets at any time will usually appreciate this.

Thirdly, analgesics may be taken prophylactically. This is most important in the elderly, when they may be fighting hard to maintain independence. Thus, the task of getting up in the morning, washing, and eating breakfast may be greatly helped by the taking of an analgesic on first waking in the morning. It is unusual for patients to get gastrointestinal side-effects from the paracetamol-containing preparations. Provided that the analgesic is not based on and does not contain aspirin or a NSAID (e.g. ibuprofen which is available without prescription), it should be safe without taking food first. Some will prefer to keep a flask of milk by the bed so that they can have a drink of milk before taking the tablet. On other occasions, activities such as doing the shopping, or even walking across the room to the toilet, can be timed to coincide with the maximum benefit obtained from drug treatment. Performance of the home exercises (pp. 8–9) should also be timed in this way.

The great advances that have been made in recent years in the treatment of pain caused by terminal cancer show that, if needed, patients can be safely treated for years with small doses of opiates without excessive side-effects. For the very old person struggling to remain independent with intractable pain from, for example, inoperable osteoarthritis of the hip, this form of therapy should be considered.

Psychological and social management

Fear

Fear may dominate the lives of many with arthritis. It has been said that 'the most important aspect of management of the rheumatic diseases is to allay the patient's fear'.[2] The inhibiting effects of fear on the low back pain patient are discussed on pp. 59–60.

People are most afraid of the unknown, and in the early stages of arthritis, the course of the illness often cannot be predicted, creating difficulties for the doctor in giving advice, and allowing the patient to fear the worst. To many patients the word 'arthritis' means using a wheelchair.[2] A future of unremitting pain and increasing disability, with loss of dignity consequent upon a perceived future of dependence upon others, particularly loved ones, makes even the most phlegmatic individual afraid. For some there is the fear that when they most need either professional or practical help, it will not be forthcoming. For others, the paramount fear is that their next movement will change their chronic nagging pain into an excruciating searing pain, or even aggravate their disability by making their arthritis worse.

Doctors have a crucial role in identifying and attempting to alleviate these fears. Firstly, an explanation of the diagnosis, and a discussion about the likely effects, is mandatory. Reassurance that only a very small number of patients require a wheelchair will be helpful. Patients must understand that the very severely disabled people seen in the waiting area at the hospital out-patient department are by definition those most needing help, and thus the 'tip of the arthritis iceberg'. Many will be suffering from a different form of arthritis. In this context, the use of the term 'osteoarthrosis', as distinct from 'osteoarthritis', may be helpful.

The importance of such counselling can be seen from the following example: 'So why am I coping now? One thing I did was to communicate with my doctors about my condition and learn all I could.' In this way fear is considerably eradicated, and anxiety lessened. 'The fact that I have knowledge and understanding about my complaint helps me to make sensible decisions based on that knowledge and stress is certainly reduced'.[3]

A consistent and supportive relationship with the doctor is vital. Once a relationship of trust has been established, intervals between appointments may be quite long, yet enable the patient to feel 'in touch'. Where it is not possible for such a relationship to be built up between the patient and a single doctor, it should be recognized that it is usually to the patient's detriment.[2]

Understanding pain

It is unlikely that a good doctor–patient relationship will develop without understanding the nature of the arthritic pain, which takes a number of forms. In acute inflammation, it may be very sharp when the joint is moved, and throb at other times. It may stop the patient from performing activities, and the fear of bringing it on further inhibits doing things. When the inflammation settles, mild pain may persist. It is the inevitability of this mild pain, day after day, which makes it increasingly difficult to bear.[2] A sudden false move brings back the sharp pain again. In the late stage of any arthritis, the grinding of the bones may be heard, giving the observer an eerie insight into what the patient must be feeling.

Long-standing pain may give rise to depression, and this is well recognized in rheumatoid arthritis.[2] Diurnal fluctuation of mood, loss of more than 6–7 kg of weight not attributed to disease activity, apathy and self-pity replacing previous interests, hopelessness, and even suicidal ideas give clues that urgent attention is needed.

Psychogenic rheumatism takes three forms: pure, in which no underlying organic disease can be identified; superimposed (functional overlay), in which an organic disease is magnified by non-organic factors; and residual (functional prolongation), in which the organic disease no longer produces the symptoms complained of.[2] In our experience, pure psychogenic rheumatism is rare. Often a fear of arthritis, multiple sclerosis or cancer magnifies an otherwise mild referred pain or sensory abnormality, often from the spine, to produce the superimposed or residual pain. A common finding is contact with, or a family history of, the condition in question.

Marital and sexual relationships

The effect of a sudden onset of disability on the spouse or other family members is explored in greater depth in Chapter 5 on stroke. With arthritis, the changes may be more gradual. Involvement of the spouse in discussions with the doctor or other members of the rehabilitation team decreases the chances of misunderstanding or manipulation by either the patient or the spouse. Arthritis affects individuals with weak marriages as well as strong ones, and the arthritis may be used as an excuse to withdraw from chores or undesired activities, including sexual ones. Conversely, the partner may be too afraid of causing pain to suggesting continuing previous activities. The consequences of either situation may be that the patient does not achieve all that otherwise would have been possible. Any substantial disability places additional strains on other members of the family, who may on occasions need both physical and emotional support. This may require a marked adjustment on the part of either or both partners. Thus the very houseproud individual with active rheumatoid arthritis may find it extremely difficult to come to terms with the need for a home help to assist with the household chores, particularly when the home help fails to meet previous very high standards. The partner may feel guilty for being unable to take on an additional role effectively.

Arthritis may impair sexual opportunity, with decreased mobility lessening the chances of meeting people, and thus of establishing sexual relationships. Physical beauty is reduced by deformed joints and sexual sparkle dimmed by chronic pain and fatigue, resulting in impairment of sexual image. Sexual drive may be reduced by mechanical difficulties, pain, the fear of pain, and the effects of medication. Sexual expression is affected by difficulties in caressing, embracing, supporting body weight, and in positioning. Involvement of the mouth, skin, genitalia, or the anal region may create additional difficulties. The presence of increased pain with morning stiffness, at the time when a man normally has maximal sexual drive, may increase frustration.[4] These problems will be felt by both partners, either of whom may seek, openly or incidentally, advice from the caring professions.

Such difficulties may not be appreciated by professional advisers, unless they are specifically looked for. When exploring this area with an individual, it is best to do so when there is plenty of time, and to approach the subject with an open question, such as: 'How does this affect your sexual relationship?'[2] If the enquiry reveals that all is not well, the sexual attitudes and behaviour before the illness began may help to define the nature of the current difficulties. Any serious arthritis is likely to give rise to pain during intercourse, but involvement of the hips or hands create the biggest difficulties. There are a number of ways in which couples having such difficulties may be helped. It is important that both partners should learn to talk to each other. Thus, one partner, not wishing to hurt the other, may abstain, and this may be misinterpreted as meaning that the partner no longer cares. When intercourse is attempted but is painful, an analgesic taken beforehand may be helpful. A hot bath or shower may also be soothing and relaxing, and participation of the partner can turn this into a type of foreplay.[2] Some people remain conservative in positioning, and may be helped by advice about the wide variety of positions which can be used. On occasions intercourse may become impossible, but many people obtain great satisfaction from stimulation of the genital organs by stroking, kissing and caressing. Others experience tremendous emotional comfort by simply lying together and enjoying the gentlest of caresses.[2] Some of these points are discussed in the Arthritis and Rheumatism Council booklet *Arthritis: Sexual Aspects and Parenthood* (see Appendix 1.1). The important point is that erosions in family harmony may be more damaging than radiological ones.[2]

Menstruation, contraception and pregnancy

When a young woman has arthritis, many different problems emerge. The practical problems of running a home are briefly outlined below. Advice may be sought about pregnancy. If more children are desired, how practical will it be to bring up an enlarged family? What will be the effect of pregnancy on the arthritis? When should the woman get pregnant, and what will be the effect on the fetus of her tablets if she is taking them at the time of conception, or during the first trimester? Will breast-feeding still be possible, and what will be the effects of treatment on the baby? If no more children are wanted, what is the best form of contraception and will the arthritis tablets interfere with the efficacy of the 'pill'?

There may be no readily available answers for all these worries. Questions about drug therapy and pregnancy or lactation are best answered following advice from the regional drug information service, which guarantees the doctor up-to-date information. The prognosis for the arthritis is best given by a consultant rheumatologist, and if such advice has not been sought, it should give some guidance as to the likely progression of the disease. Another factor to bear in mind is the degree of support likely to be available from spouse, parents, in-laws and friends or neighbours. Common-sense advice has to be given in the light of these factors and the depth of desire to have a baby. There is a definite risk of a postpartum flare in rheumatoid arthritis. The practical difficulties of bringing up young children must militate against having a large family, and 3–4 years' gap between children is probably advisable.

Arthritic fingers may have difficulties in inserting a contraceptive cap, and also in coping with sanitary towels and tampons. Intrauterine contraceptive devices may encourage a heavy menstrual flow. These factors may favour the contraceptive pill, as periods are usually lightened when the pill is taken.

Group therapy

Several centres have described group meetings (see also pp. 103, 128–30). Such groups are usually supportive, and frequently are related to centres where people are treated as inpatients, where staff can interact informally, and help to rebuild self-confidence. One group is described which met as outpatients on a weekly basis for 8 months. When the group meetings concluded, 3 of the 14 patients suffered a relapse of their arthritis.[2] Thus it is important to note that psychological and emotional factors do seem to play a part, even though the evidence appears anecdotal.

Other groups may be formed by patients themselves, without therapeutic input. Thus the Northwick Park Arthritis and Rheumatism Club is organized by a committee of members and aims to foster a greater understanding of the causes and treatment of the rheumatic diseases, for sufferers and their relatives. It also promotes support for those within the club, encourages self-help with problems, and provides a social meeting-place for members and their guests. Coach outings, bingo, film shows and parties or concerts all help to brighten up the day for members and friends, with meetings at monthly intervals.

Many branches of Arthritis Care are now offering informal counselling to patients in, or after discharge from hospital, and patients have the chance to join the local branch.

Some patients maintain their zest for life through their leisure activities, such as the champion angler shown in Figure 1.3.

General points

Some patients, either because of their stoic nature, or through a desire not to waste the doctor's time do not ask about, or discuss, the different aspects of their disease. Some may do so if the doctor asks leading questions. Others come with an enormous list of problems, usually not written down. Here the difficulty is in deciding which problems require speedy solutions. 'What

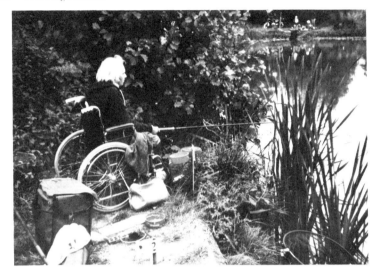

Fig. 1.3   Despite severe deforming rheumatoid arthritis this man remains a champion angler, illustrating the importance of orienting rehabilitation to the development or maintenance of activities

bothers you most?' is often a valuable starting point. A written list at the next visit often enables the limited available time to be spent where there is the greatest concern.

The two most important points to emphasize are firstly, that many of those who suffer from the different forms of arthritis do not become severely disabled, and are able to continue to lead relatively normal lives. Secondly, if in spite of the many different forms of medical or surgical treatment, arthritis progresses and leads to increasing disability, there are still many ways in which the caring professions can help.

Environmental management

The environment in which the arthritic person lives has already been emphasized in the social assessment. For some, the help that can be given in their daily lives appears more useful than their tablets, particularly if patients are prone to side-effects, or have aggressive disease. Life may be dominated by the presence of steps or stairs, or the absence of a downstairs toilet. For convenience this section will be divided into three areas, that of the nature and siting of the home, adapting the home, and equipment to facilitate personal independence. To some degree, all these factors are interdependent.

The site and nature of the arthritis is the important factor in determining what advice we should be giving people with arthritis (Table 1.5). Those with a rapidly progressive polyarthropathy (e.g. aggressive rheumatoid arthritis) will need to consider all these areas. Those with mild osteoarthritis of only one or two joints of the hands will not be concerned about the site of the home in relation to other facilities. No adaptations are needed, but the provision of one or two gadgets to facilitate writing, or to help with opening bottles or jars, or even to turn on the gas cooker, may transform the life of a writer, or an old person living on his or her own. If, however, the arthritis is affecting the shoulder joints alone, and the provision of modified clothing and/or aids has not enabled dressing to be performed independently, it may be the close proximity of a friend or relative who is prepared to come in daily to help with dressing which will be the determining factor. Where the large joints of the lower limbs are predominantly affected, the loss of mobility will be the key handicap. A similar loss of mobility may be found consequent to severe low back pain, particularly if the pain is referred to the legs. Here, the site of the home in relation to friends, relatives, shops, general practitioner's surgery, or even the local bingo hall, may be the important factor.

Nature and siting of the home

As families grow up and move away from the home, people see the advantage of moving into a smaller home, which they think will suit them for their retirement needs. They see this as a normal pattern in the life cycle. People with arthritis can be encouraged to make such considerations. It makes sense to make the same decisions as other people do, but in their situation, to consider making them earlier. People who can be helped in this way include those with rheumatoid arthritis whose disease appears to be progressive and those with osteoarthritis involving the large joints of the legs. Whilst joint replacement surgery can help many people, it should not be relied upon to solve all the problems of decreasing mobility, particularly if there is multiple joint involvement, or if old age is approaching.

Regrettably, many people do not make the decision when they are in a position to make a big difference to their lives. If people have not moved by their mid-70s, they are unlikely to summon up the energy to do so. This may result in an old person living by him- or herself in the old family home which is in a poor state of decoration and repair with too much furniture and a large untended garden.

Whilst such problems may be at their most dramatic in the very old, many will suffer from isolation. Although a relatively small number of people handicapped from arthritis are housebound, many more will be unable to

Table 1.5 Environmental management of arthritis – some illustrations

Skeletal impairment	Disabilities	Possible solutions	Overall handicap
Hand and wrists Loss of dexterity Poor grip Deformity (?)	Personal hygiene Dressing Eating Knobs/locks etc. Writing/typing	Closomat (automatic self-cleaning lavatory) Velcro: front fastening Wide-handled cutlery Levers, key holders Word processing	*Difficulties* Work/housework Making/maintaining relationships Shopping Communication
Shoulders Inability to reach	Difficulty with high cupboards, eating, dressing, combing hair, driving	Advice on positioning Long-handled cutlery Long-handled comb Long-handled gear lever	*Losses* Dignity Body image Independence Friends (social isolation)
Hip and knees Immobility	Difficulty getting up from chair and toilet Difficulty with stairs and walking	Chair blocks Personal chair Raised toilet seat Adaptations: lift/elevator Walking aids Independence on one floor (?) move house	
Ankles and feet Immobility	Difficulty in walking	Chiropody Special shoes	

(Based on definitions from World Health Organisation 1980)

walk 100 yards, and this may be far shorter than the distance to the nearest shop. The bus stop may be further away, even supposing that the individual will be able to climb on to the bus. Many will have to entertain at home, and dislike being dependent on friends coming to see them as it affects the type of relationship.[5]

If people make early plans, there is a better chance of their being able to make the best compromise between the following factors: close proximity to long-standing friends and neighbours; nearness of shops; attractive bungalow or ground-floor flat which is affordable and has easy access; and for the more severely affected individual, the facility to convert the residence to wheelchair-adapted accommodation if needed. For those in council property, early application for a transfer to ground-floor accommodation is encouraged in view of the shortage of suitable housing.

Adaptations to the home

Much can be done to help arthritic people inside and outside the home. Substituting ramps for steps, both inside and out may make an enormous difference. Extra banisters or rails facilitate climbing stairs or steps. This is important to people whose only toilet is upstairs and who spend most of their time downstairs. Strategically placed grab rails facilitate movement around the house and may particularly help people getting on and off the toilet, in and out of the bath, or at difficult corners, particularly on staircases.

Difficulties in managing stairs create the greatest distress for many people. Many will have osteoarthritis of hips or knees, and will be elderly, and so are likely to have multiple impairments, such as difficulties with their balance. When simpler measures have failed a number of alternatives are available. The provision of an easily accessible downstairs toilet is one of the most worthwhile adaptations, but needs to be planned in advance. This is most useful as part of a strategy so that, if stairs become impossible in the long term, independence may be maintained by living on the ground floor, usually by converting a downstairs room into a bedroom. In an emergency, a downstairs commode or chemical toilet may suffice. On occasions, the provision of an elevator (Fig. 1.4), or more rarely a lift, may enable the individual to remain in his or her own home.

Whilst many with arthritis are able to move around the home, their mobility outside the house may be very restricted and the use of a wheelchair for outdoors should be considered more frequently. It is mentioned here, as the provision of a suitably wide door, front or back, may greatly facilitate getting out, and even enable gardening to be continued.

The kitchen is another area where much suffering can be avoided with

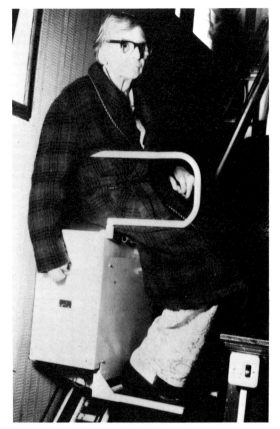

Fig. 1.4   Use of elevator to avoid having to walk up and down stairs

careful planning. Where possible, the height of the kitchen surfaces should be modified to enable work to be done sitting, and surfaces should be made continuous at the same height (see p. 13). Many people have found a swivel tap at the side of a shallow sink invaluable.

These adaptations are best provided following a home assessment from an occupational therapist, usually from the social services department, but sometimes from the local hospital (ideally one specializing in helping people with arthritis, and working with the rheumatology team).

Aids or equipment for independent living

There is an almost unlimited supply of equipment available for people suffering from arthritis. Leaflets from the Arthritis and Rheumatism Council (see Appendix 1.1) can be recommended for anyone who has arthritis and *Your Home and your Rheumatism* should be available in waiting rooms of hospitals, surgeries and social service departments. Various aids are listed in Table 1.6, and illustrate the enormous potential to help people in this way.

When people initially need an aid it may be the first time that they are confronted with the reality that their arthritis is going to be, for them, a crippling disease. Some, therefore, decline the assistance that an aid would bring, as its significance is too painful. It may be seen as a stigma of disability.[2] This is understandable, and it may be difficult to decide when encouragement should become more persuasive. If it is certain that they will become more independent thanks to the aid, then they should be encouraged to use it. On occasions it is helpful to point out that the use of the aid may help the arthritis by taking the strain off the joint (see section on joint protection, above).

Although many aids are readily available commercially, it is recommended that the use of an aid is discussed with an occupational therapist who is experienced in advising people with arthritis. A number of centres modelled for the most part on the Disabled Living Foundation in London have been set up, where both professional groups and individuals are welcomed to view aids or equipment for disabled people. Everything from powered self-operated wheelchairs to adapted telephones, from bottle openers to shoe horns, is available for customers to try for themselves with expert advice on hand. Details are given in Appendix 1.2.

Before discussing different types of equipment, it must be emphasized that making full use of modern gadgets can make an enormous difference, as is illustrated in Table 1.7. Certain types of aids are most suited to arthritis of specific joints, and will be considered separately.

Feet and footwear

Numerous conditions give rise to deformity of the feet and there are many different ways to help people with such deformities.[6] For the purposes of illustration, an approach to the problems of patients suffering from rheumatoid arthritis will be discussed. In an ideal world, all patients with rheumatoid arthritis should have their feet carefully examined and given attention by a chiropodist early in the course of the disease.

The importance of wearing lace-up shoes is stressed, and avoiding slip-on shoes as these will nearly always either be too tight and compress the forefoot, or too loose and allow the foot to slip around in the shoe. Trauma to the

Table 1.6   Some aids or equipment useful to people with arthritis

Difficulty	Aid
Opening doors	Lever handles
Opening locks	Long key holders
	Use skewer as lever for mortice keys
Turning on lights	Cord pull
	Rocker switches at suitable height
Getting in and out of chairs	Adapt chair for personal use (suitable height, solid arm rests)
	Ejector seats
Writing	Magnetic board to hold paper
	Help grip with padding to widen grip of pencil
Picking things up	Pick-up tongs
Carrying	Long-handled plastic holders
	Trolley/shopping basket on wheels
Using the telephone	Padded pencils for dialling
	Push-button phone (see Table 1.7)
	Direct line to operator
	Light-weight receiver holder/amplifier
In the kitchen	Lever-type swivel taps
	Tap turner
	Multipurpose clamp for switches and dials (Fig 1.7)
	See-through saucepans with widened handles
Opening tins and jars	Wall tin opener/fixed bottle opener on wall
Carrying heavy saucepan	Continuous level surface between sink and cooker
	Swivel tap on side of sink
	Use perforated wire basket or spoon for straining
Eating and drinking	Use padded handles for cutlery, especially knives
	Cutlery can be angled
	Use insulated mugs/cups
Ironing	Adjustable-height ironing board – iron sitting
Using the bathroom/toilet	Board across bath
	Fitted shower units
	Portable plastic bidet
	Toilet handrails
	Raised seat
	Tongs for holding and releasing paper after wiping
	Push-button flush operated by hand or foot
	Closomat
Dressing	Avoid hooks and zips
	Use velcro
	Gutter or double gutter for stockings or tights
	Elastic laces for tie-up shoes
	Long-handled shoe horn

Table 1.7   Modern conveniences useful for people with arthritis

Self-cleaning oven – oven and burners in separate compartments

Slow cookers

Microwave ovens

Front-loading upright freezer in kitchen

Electric food processors

Light-weight carpet sweepers

Light-weight cellular blankets/duvets

Washing machines (or spin and tumble dryer)

Fitted shower units

Plastic portable bidets

Modern telephones – memory, redial, no hands conversation

---

foot can thus be avoided with well fitting lace-up shoes, particularly noting the importance of avoiding pressure on the toes by pointed shoes.

Pain often occurs at the metatarsophalangeal joints, when the metatarsal protective fat pad (which often thins with age) moves anteriorly, putting pressure on the exposed metatarsal heads. This is particularly distressing where the metatarsophalangeal joints are painful and deformed consequent to arthritis. Soft insoles to cushion the metatarsal heads can be bought commercially, or may be provided by a chiropodist who may have the facility to make such supports to measure. Often supports are discarded by patients who feel they create pressure inside the shoe. This may be corrected by the prescription of extra-depth shoes (Fig. 1.5); one variety is on the market and may be provided by an orthotist following prescription in hospital. Such shoes are particularly helpful for forefoot problems, are light-weight and have soft uppers. These shoes are not everybody's idea of fashion but look more normal than the old classical black 'made to measure' shoes. By and large, extra-depth shoes are prescribed more often now than John Locke shoes (made to measure on adapted standard lasts) and Drushoes, which are mouldable thermoplastic shoes, and may be moulded to shape the individual's foot.

All special footwear has to be prescribed by hospital medical staff, and is supplied by orthotists who are either employed or contracted by the hospital to provide this service. Chiropody is available under the National Health Service (NHS) to children under 16, women over 60 and men over 65, all registered disabled people and expectant mothers. Patients outside these

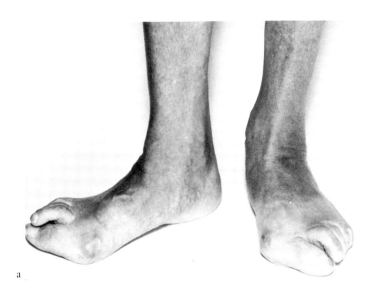

a

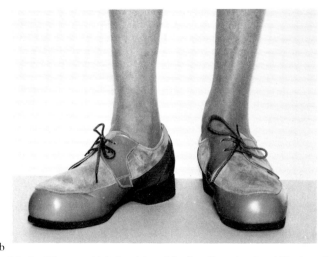

b

Fig. 1.5a,b   Rheumatoid deformities of the feet. Functional mobility is maintained by the use of extra-depth shoes, which are visually acceptable to many patients

categories who regularly attend an NHS hospital that has a chiropodist are also entitled to treatment. Chiropodists not only advise on appropriate supports or footwear, but are often in a position to make moulded insoles to suit individual needs. A domiciliary chiropody service is available in most health districts for housebound patients who fulfil the above criteria.

Whilst most forefoot difficulties can be coped with by wearing extra-depth shoes, mid- and hindfoot problems may require made to measure shoes, which are approximately five times as expensive as the shoes mentioned above.

Careful attention to feet is most worthwhile as these relatively simple measures may transform an individual's life, making walking a pleasure again. The indications for surgery are outside the remit of this chapter, but surgery may be highly successful when these measures fail or are inappropriate.

Large joints of the lower limbs

The strain taken by the lower limbs when getting out of a low chair, or off a low toilet, is enormous. Not only does this strain potentially increase the damage to already deranged joints, but the movement is usually extremely painful. Help may be inappropriately obtained by putting extra strain on the hands, wrists and elbows. The most important principle is that arthritic individuals should have chairs of their own. These can be modified to suit them. The height of the chair can most easily be raised by blocks placed under the feet of the chair, and these can be supplied by the social services department. Strong, well padded arm rests are essential to support the arms during sitting, and for ease of getting up. Ejector seats may be invaluable for the carefully selected individual, and should only be obtained after trying out the chair with an occupational therapist.

Similarly, it is much easier to get up off a toilet which has a high seat. This is particularly important for the elderly person on diuretics for hypertension or fluid retention, or who has frequency of micturition for any reason. Postural oedema is often seen in the severely disabled individual who may be forced into a predominantly sedentary existence. Clearly the logical treatment for this type of postural oedema would be elastic tights or stockings, but these may be impossible to put on with arthritic hands, and often no one is available to help.

One other important principle is to avoid standing if it is painful (see Fig. 2.7) and unnecessary. Thus ironing can be done sitting if the ironing board is at a suitable height, as may many other kitchen chores if the kitchen surfaces are at the appropriate level. Many elderly patients with back pain and

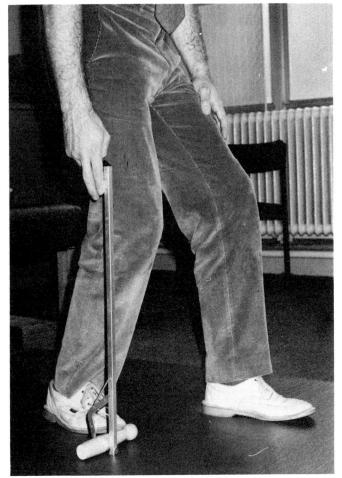

Fig. 1.6   Use of a 'helping hand' to lift fallen objects without excessive flex-ion of the spine, hips and knees

arthritis of large joints in the legs find a 'helping hand' assists in retrieving fallen objects from the floor without bending back or legs (Fig. 1.6).

Arthritis of the shoulder

Loss of function of the shoulder results in reduced function of the whole arm. The commonest causes of shoulder pain relate to problems arising from the support structures of the shoulder joint, particularly the rotator cuff. Involvement in rheumatoid arthritis, however, does occur and can be devastating in combination with arthritis in other joints in the arms. Osteoarthritis of the shoulders is seen in older people. When dressing, it is usually easiest to put the arm with the worst shoulder into the sleeve first, and when undressing to take the arm with the worst shoulder out of the sleeve last. The loss of reach can affect getting the hands behind the back (for example, when fastening bras and washing the back). Help can be obtained by using long-, and sometimes angled handles for cutlery, combs and scrubbing brushes etc. (Tables 1.5 and 1.6).

Arthritis of the small joints of the hands

Involvement of the small joints of the hands is usual in rheumatoid arthritis, and is seen not infrequently in osteoarthritis when it may commonly affect the carpometacarpal joint at the base of the thumb. The result is weakness of grip, which is particularly marked in rheumatoid arthritis. Help can be given by increasing the size of the object being gripped. Good examples are key holders, pens and pencils, cutlery etc. Converting knobs into handles or long levers whenever possible is useful (e.g. taps). Multipurpose clamps with spring-loaded rods which conform to the shape of the object being gripped are often useful for awkward knobs (Fig. 1.7). British Gas provide a free advisory service for their customers.

Many articles of clothing are suitable and many clothes can be easily adapted. When button hooks are unhelpful, velcro fastening is a good substitute for buttons, as well as for zips. There is a full range of clothing specially designed for wheelchair users.

Help with sleep

Anything that facilitates a good night's rest is to be encouraged. Heavy blankets are particularly uncomfortable. However, light-weight cellular blankets, or continental quilts (duvets) are generally found to be very acceptable. Duvets have the added advantage that beds do not need to be made.

Helping with the consequences of arthritis

Mobility (including wheelchairs and driving)

The facilitation of transfers has already been referred to. Chartered physiotherapists help people to walk through maintaining muscle strength and a

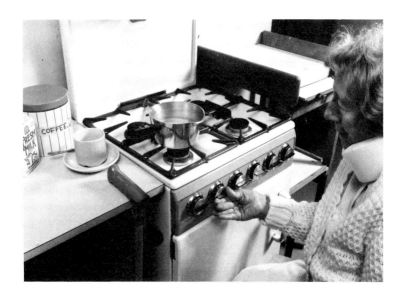

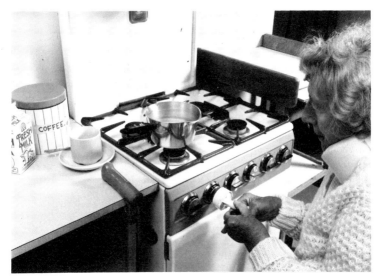

Fig. 1.7 Use of a multipurpose clamp with spring-loaded rods to help a woman with weak deformed rheumatoid hands use her gas cooker

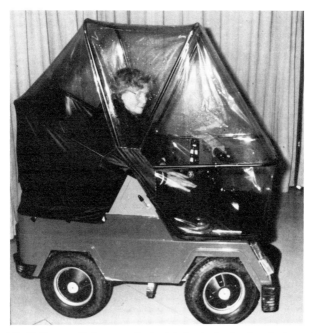

Fig. 1.8   Self-controlled powered wheelchair obtained privately (sometimes making use of the Motability Scheme – see p. 141) enables a woman with gross osteoarthrosis of the spine and knees to maintain a social life outside her home

maximal range of movement of the leg joints, and/or easing the strain on joints with sticks or elbow crutches. The elimination of steps and stairs where needed is very helpful. If these measures are unsuccessful, mobility inside the house may be maintained with a struggle, but the individual may become housebound. A wheelchair for outdoor use may be most helpful. Although the current NHS provision of self-operated powered chairs for outdoor use is inadequate, chairs or tricycles (Figs 1.8 and 8.5) can be obtained privately. For those in receipt of the mobility allowance, various schemes are available to help finance such a purchase. The need for a wheelchair for indoor use is very rare considering the prevalence of arthritis of the lower limbs. The fear of requiring a wheelchair has already been noted, and the refusal to use one is a well recognized defence mechanism. It must be stressed, however, that the isolation of a person because he or she is housebound is a high price to pay, and may contribute to depression. The many ways people can travel in spite of their disability are further discussed in the Appendix to Chapter 5.

Driving should be encouraged as it enables patients to maintain their independence. An automatic car with power steering has many advantages, but a manual car can be adapted by the provision of a longer gear lever, or a different knob. Door handles can be changed, steering wheels and hand-brakes adapted, and other individual problems attended to. Where a car needs many adaptations it is often necessary for the patient to take a number of driving lessons. These can be booked through the Disabled Driver branch of the British School of Motoring. If the patient is a driver by trade he or she can apply to the Training Commission for the necessary adaptations to be done. If the patient is a social driver then he or she should apply through the DHSS who keep a register of local garages which do conversions.

Application for exemption from wearing seat belts is obtained by writing, together with a medical certificate, to: Department of Transport, Disability Unit, 2 Marsham Street, London SW1P 3EP.

Employment

If a patient is unable, through disability, to continue his or her current employment and needs to seek alternative and more suitable work, or requires rehabilitation and retraining, he or she should apply to the Disablement Resettlement Officer for an interview either at the district hospital, or at the local Job Centre (see pp. 61 and 132–3).

Gardening

Many useful adapted tools are available for the keen gardener. Kneeling should be avoided. Electric or petrol-driven lawn mowers are an advantage and the greenhouse level of work is ideal. Information on suitable tools can be obtained from an occupational therapist.

THE OVERALL HANDICAP

Words are not often used to describe the deepest feelings people have about their handicaps. The most easily recognized is that of social isolation (Table 1.5), but equally painful are the loss of dignity consequent to the need for help from equipment or people, and the loss of self-image as beautiful hands become deformed and special shoes replace high heels.

The frustration of difficulties experienced day after day becomes harder to live with, and the inability to fill one's 'proper role in life', by earning a wage or doing the chores, adds to the inner agony.

Discussion of these difficulties, particularly with others who share them, helps. The objective of professional helpers is to strive continually to find roles or tasks which continue to allow self-fulfilment for those with arthritis.

THE VOLUNTARY SECTOR

Whilst the use of the small group or club has already been referred to, a large number of groups exist to promote support for sufferers from the rheumatic diseases and research into their causes and treatment. Organizations give support to people suffering from specific conditions, including systemic lupus erythematosus, scleroderma, juvenile chronic arthritis and osteoporosis, in addition to the previously mentioned National Ankylosing Spondylitis Society (see Chapter 14).

The two major charities are the Arthritis and Rheumatism Council (ARC), and Arthritis Care. Some millions of pounds are raised annually by the ARC for the foundation of research institutes, providing research grants, and funding academic posts in our medical schools. In addition, the education committee of the ARC publishes many booklets which have been of great value to patients and professionals alike; these are listed in Appendix 1.1.

Arthritis Care, on the other hand, promotes the welfare of those with arthritis in different ways. Its paper *Arthritis News* is published quarterly and contains articles about gardening, cookery and aids or equipment suitable for people with arthritis. It also provides information about the treatment of arthritis and services for those suffering from its effects. In addition it has a problem page in which a consultant rheumatologist answers readers' questions. Arthritis Care also has a few holiday centres and 10 self-catering family holiday units, a residential home, a homework division for the housebound, and a scholarship fund for young people disabled with arthritis.[2] The supportive role of the local branch of Arthritis Care for individuals with arthritis is expanding and is referred to above. Fact sheets describing the work of Arthritis Care are available (Appendix 1.1).

The work of many other charities is relevant to people with arthritis, and some of these are listed in Chapter 14.

CONCLUSION

This chapter outlines the various forms of help available to people with arthritis, the commonest of the disabling conditions. Many areas which are often neglected are emphasized, such as the physical, environmental, psychological and social aspects of management.

For people with mild impairments, the handicap may be greater than needed through unnecessary fear of pain, disability or dependence on others.

For those with multiple impairments, the handicap may be devastating, and includes the indignity of relying on other people or equipment for one's personal independence, constant pain limiting all aspects of life, loss of self-image as joints become deformed and smart shoes impossible to wear and social isolation consequent to immobility.

Doctors, together with the other caring professions, have an important role to play in alleviating fear, controlling pain, encouraging a positive attitude to disability, and ensuring that patients get the help they require to lead the fullest life possible.

REFERENCES

1. Journal of the Royal College of Physicians (1986), Physical disability in 1986 and beyond – a report of the Royal College of Physicians, *J. Roy. Coll. Phys. (Lond)*; **20**: 161–94.
2. Woolf D., ed. (1981), Rehabilitation in the rheumatic diseases, *Clin. Rheum. Dis.*; **7**.
3. Fox C. (1986), Coping with arthritis, *Arthr. Rheum. Council Magazine*; **66**: 7–8.
4. Hamilton A. (1981), Sexual problems in arthritis and allied conditions, *Int. Rehab. Med.*; **3**: 38–42.
5. Buchanan J. M., Chamberlain M. A. (1978), *Survey of the Mobility of the Disabled in an Urban Environment*, London, Royal Association for Disability and Rehabilitation.
6. Hughes, J. (1983), *Footwear and Foot Care for Adults*, London, Disabled Living Foundation.

FURTHER READING

Chamberlain M. A., Care G., Harfield B. (1982), Physiotherapy and osteoarthritis of the knees, *Int. Rehab. Med.*; **4**: 101–6.
Scott J. T. ed (1986), *Copeman's Textbook of the Rheumatic Diseases*, 6th edn, London, Churchill Livingstone.
World Health Organization (1980), *International Classification of Impairments, Disabilities and Handicaps*, Geneva, WHO.

Appendix 1.1

Information suitable for people with arthritis

The following literature has been written for patients with rheumatic diseases and is available free of charge from the Arthritis and Rheumatism Council for Research, 41 Eagle Street, London WC1R 4AR (bulk orders are accepted from doctors and other professional carers – postage will be charged).

Handbooks

1. Osteoarthritis explained
2. Rheumatoid arthritis explained
3. Pain in the neck
4. Backache
5. Ankylosing spondylitis
6. Gout
7. Lupus (SLE)
8. When your child has arthritis
9. Introducing arthritis
10. Your home and your rheumatism
11. Are you sitting comfortably?
12. Arthritis: sexual aspects and parenthood

Leaflets

1. Polymyalgia rheumatica (PMR)
2. A new hip joint
3. Tennis elbow
4. Choosing shoes
5. Alternative medicine

Information sheets

1. Allergy
2. Diet and arthritis
3. Weather
4. Exercise

The following fact sheets are available from Arthritis Care, 6, Grosvenor Crecent, London SW1X 7ER:

1. Arthritis care
2. Pain killers and anti-inflammatory drugs
3. Physiotherapy
4. Sources of help
5. Basic reading
6. Equipment and aids for disability
7. Diet
8. Residential accommodation
9. How we can help your patient
10. Money (income and expenditure of Arthritis Care)

Appendix 1.2

Disabled living centres

Aid centres offering a fully comprehensive service

Belfast	Prosthetic Orthotic and Aids Service, Musgrave Park Hospital, Stockman's Lane, Belfast BT9 7JB. Tel: 0232 669501
Birmingham	Disabled Living Centre, 260 Broad Street, Birmingham B1 2HF. Tel: 021 643 0980
Caerphilly	Aid and Information Centre, Wales Council for the Disabled, Caerbragdy Industrial Estate, Bedwas Road, Caerphilly, Mid Glamorgan CF8 3SL. Tel: 0222 887325/6/7
Cardiff	The Demonstration Aids Centre, The Lodge, Rookwood Hospital, Llandaff, Cardiff, South Glamorgan CF5 2YN. Tel: 0222 566281
Edinburgh	South Lothian Disabled Living Centre, Astley Ainsley Hospital, Grange Loan, Edinburgh EH9 2HL. Tel: 031 447 6271, ext. 241
Leeds	The William Merritt Disabled Living Centre, St Mary's Hospital, Greenhill Road, Leeds LS12 3QE. Tel: 0532 793140
Leicester	TRAIDS (Trent Region Aids, Information and Demonstration Service), 76 Clarendon Park Road, Leicester LE2 3AD. Tel: 0533 700747/8
Liverpool	Merseyside Aids Centre, Youens Way, East Prescott Road, Liverpool L14 2EP. Tel: 051 228 9221
London	Disabled Living Foundation, Aids and Equipment Centre, 380–384 Harrow Road, London W9 2HU. Tel: 01 289 6111
Manchester	Disabled Living Services, Disabled Living Centre, Redbank House, 4 St Chads Street, Cheetham, Manchester M8 8QA. Tel: 061 832 3678
Newcastle upon Tyne	Newcastle upon Tyne Council for the Disabled, The Dene Centre, Castles Farm Road, Newcastle upon Tyne, NE3 1PH. Tel: 091 2840480
Nottingham	Nottingham Resource Centre for the Disabled, Lenton Business Centre, Lenton Boulevard, Nottingham NG7 2BY. Tel: 0602 420 391
Sheffield	Sheffield Independent Living Centre, 108 The Moor, Sheffield, S1 4DP. Tel: 0742 737025
Southampton	Southampton Aids and Equipment Centre, Southampton General Hospital, Tremona Road, Southampton SO9 4XY. Tel: 0703 777222, ext. 3414/3233

Stockport   Aids/Assessment Unit, Stockport Area Health Authority, St Thomas's Hospital, Shawheath, Stockport SK3 8BL. Tel: 061 419 4476

Swindon   The Swindon Centre for Disabled Living, The Hawthorn Centre, Cricklade Road, Swindon, Wilts SA2 1AF. Tel: 0793 643966

Aid centres offering a limited service

Blackpool   Disabled Living Centre, 8 Queen Street, Blackpool, Lancs FY1 1PD. Tel: 0253 21084, ext. 1

Dudley   Dudley Disabled Living Centre, 1 St Giles Street, Netherton, Dudley DY2 0PR. Tel: 0384 55433

Huddersfield Disabled Living Centre, Silver Court, Silver Street, Huddersfield HD5 9AG. Tel: 0484 518809

Macclesfield Centre for Disabled Living, Macclesfield District General Hospital, Macclesfield, Cheshire SK10 3BL. Tel: 0625 21000

Middlesbrough Dept. of Rehabilitation, Middlesbrough General Hospital, Ayresome Green Lane, Middlesbrough, Cleveland TS5 5AZ. Tel: 0642 813133, ext. 158

Paisley   Disabled Centre for Independent Living, Community Services Centre, Paisley. Tel: 041 887 0597

Portsmouth   Disabled Living Centre, Prince Albert Road, Eastney, Portsmouth PO4 9HR. Tel: 0705 737174

Further information is avilable from:
The Disabled Living Centre Council, TRAIDS, 76 Clarendon Park Road, Leicester LE2 3AD. Tel: 0533 700747–8

2

Spinal pain

Andrew Frank and Jacqueline E. Hills

INTRODUCTION

This chapter is not designed to review all the facets of the management of spinal pain, neither is it designed to look comprehensively at its causes. The evidence that much idiopathic low back pain is due to mechanical stress on spinal structures is outlined.

The major emphasis of this chapter is on the effects of postural and ergonomic factors in everyday life, and how they may be modified. Whilst many physical and drug regimens are outlined in some detail, the main objective is to describe how people may be helped to avoid stress on the spine on a day-to-day basis. This helps to lessen the severity of pain at any moment in time, and to reduce the risk of a recurrence of pain.

Because of the individual nature of the condition it is impossible to give dogmatic guidelines about management. The chapter sections outline those areas of management which experience suggests help the vast majority of patients, but there will always be some individuals who will not conform to the average picture.

THE SPINE

The spine is extremely complex, constituting 139 joints and numerous bursae, as well as a vast number of ligaments and muscles comprising support structures. Symptoms may arise from any of these structures. Pain, a subjective symptom, is the cardinal feature of spinal disorders. There are no objective physical signs or laboratory investigations to help physicians to confirm, in their own minds, the precise cause and severity of the pain, and so evaluation is difficult. It is not surprising, therefore, that spinal pain remains an enigma. Doctors trained to intervene in well understood disease processes may have difficulty in coping with spinal pain of uncertain cause, with consequent difficulty in inspiring confidence in the patient, who may therefore seek help from heterodox practitioners.

A further complicating feature of the spine is the compartmentalization into the neck, thorax and the low back. Whilst this is eminently sensible on anatomical grounds, it hinders a realistic approach to treatment. The anatomical differences are important. The cervical spine has a low weight-bearing capacity, and its facet and atlantoaxial joints are specifically designed to facilitate mobility. The thoracic spine is splinted by the costovertebral joints, which perhaps helps to explain the decreased frequency of symptoms arising from the thoracic spine. The lumbar spine is primarily designed to take the weight of the upper part of the body, with less facility for movement. All sections of the spine contain the spinal canal, and it is the size and shape of this canal which may be a key factor in determining who will suffer symptoms from degenerative spinal disease.

EPIDEMIOLOGY

The scale of the problem is frightening. There are no good recent epidemiological data on the frequency of cervical pain. Low back pain has been studied in some detail, although the limitations of these studies are beyond the scope of this chapter, and are reviewed in detail elsewhere. It has been estimated that 2.2 million people see their general practitioner for low back pain annually, of whom 10–20% will be referred to a hospital. In 1982 approximately 63 000 people were admitted to hospital with spinal pain (only 3% cervical) in England, Scotland and Wales. Probably less than 10 000 operations are performed on the lumbar spine (see Fig. 2.1).

Low back pain is a relatively small cause of severe permanent disability. Figures vary from 34–52 per 1000 people with significant morbidity from low back pain, of which only 0.2–4 per 1000 are severely disabled.[2] Whilst the difficulties in collecting such data limit their value, the point remains that the proportion of back pain sufferers who become permanently severely disabled is very small.

Nonetheless, consequences for employment and the provision of health care are enormous. Back pain is one of the commonest causes of inability to work through sickness, with 33.3 million workings days lost in Britain in 1982–3 greater than for either coronary heart disease or bronchitis, and more than six times the number of working days lost through industrial stoppages. It has been calculated that the cost to the economy exceeded £156 million in 1982,[1] and such calculations ignore the effects on the individual, the family, and the problems of litigation.

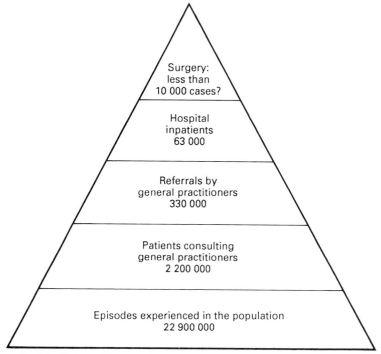

Fig. 2.1 Estimated impact of back pain over the course of a 12-month period

CAUSES OF LOW BACK PAIN – WHEN ARE INVESTIGATIONS NEEDED?

Over 90% of all episodes of low back pain may be considered idiopathic. The cause is thought to arise from the disc, the facet joints, or other supporting structures of the spine. It is on this group that this chapter will concentrate. The exclusion of serious systemic illnesses is beyond the scope of this chapter. The management of scoliosis in children and adolescents requires the expertise of an experienced orthopaedic surgeon. Metabolic bone disease will probably give a more generalized pattern of bone pain, and osteomalacia must be considered in people of Asian origin as it is eminently treatable. Infections such as tuberculosis (except in immigrant communities), brucellosis and osteomyelitis are rare, and usually associated with systemic illness. Neoplastic disease is usually secondary. In women, a gynaecological cause must be borne in mind. Although such patients are rare in a back clinic, an increase in pain in association with menstruation warrants a pelvic examination. Involvement of the lumbar spine is rare in rheumatoid arthritis, although cervical involvement is frequent, and ankylosing spondylitis is discussed on pp. 3–6.

The clinical features of the many conditions which may present with spinal pain are described in the standard texts, and will not be discussed further here. The features of spinal stenosis and hypermobility have recently been reviewed.[2] The important judgements that have to be made by the clinician relate to the necessity for investigations to exclude serious underlying illness, and to provide guidance for the management of the idiopathic spinal condition.

As low back pain is such a frequent presenting symptom, common presentations should be recognized in order to spot the rare patient with other pathology. Idiopathic low back pain usually presents in several ways, the commonest being of discomfort or pain across the low back, and sometimes it may be more severe on one or other side. Sometimes the pain is predominantly unilateral, and often refers into the buttock of the affected side. More rarely the pain may be felt in the midline. Leg pain is also a common presentation and may be difficult to diagnose unless a careful history is taken, which usually defines the pain as arising from or radiating to the buttock or back. Well localized pain arising from other sites should be treated with a degree of suspicion.

X-rays of the appropriate part of the spine are indicated during the first episode of spinal pain if symptoms are atypical, are not improving after 3 weeks, are associated with features of disease elswhere in the body, or when manipulative treatment is being planned. Before the age of 26, x-rays are indicated, looking for evidence of congenital abnormalities such as cervical ribs, fused vertebrae, spondylolisis or spondylolisthesis, and to exclude ankylosing spondylitis. The sudden onset of spinal symptoms over the age of 45 also warrants investigation.[3] In Asian immigrants, tuberculosis or metabolic bone disease may present at any age. Tuberculosis will classically involve the upper lumber vertebrae, whilst mechanical back pain usually involves the fourth and fifth lumbar segments. The presence of generalized spinal pain or tenderness warrants investigation to exclude infectious, malignant or metabolic bone disease. For infection or malignancy, the erythrocyte sedimentation rate is probably the most useful screening test, but this is not infallible and it may be normal even in the presence of carcinoma or multiple myeloma. Pain arising from the thoracic spine should always be investigated.

It is important to realize that there is usually a poor correlation between symptoms and radiological changes, particularly disc degeneration, although the correlation is closer in subjects with severe degenerative changes involving several levels. It is best to consider degenerative changes on x-ray as part of the ageing process, and many patients are reassured to find that their pain is not due to a disease as such.

Repeated episodes of spinal pain which do not vary in character or site from previous occasions do not require further investigation. A change in character or site of the pain, particularly in the later years, should be investigated. Where there is a strong suspicion of tumour, such as in a person with generalized bone pain and a history of previous malignancy, discussion with a radiologist may result in a bone scan being performed.

The presence of persisting neurological deficit is almost always an indication for a specialist opinion, as there may be a surgically remediable lesion, e.g. a disc, spinal stenosis, or other pathology. Very rarely, severe unremitting back pain (without leg pain) may require surgery.

PRECIPITATING FACTORS FOR SPINAL PAIN

Lower spine

There are a number of epidemiological studies looking at factors which may precipitate low back pain. Only those which may influence management are discussed here. The following six factors have been shown to be associated with sickness absence due to low back pain: physically heavy work; static work postures; frequent bending and twisting; lifting and forceful movements; repetitive work; and vibrations. All increase the load on the spine. Psychological aspects such as monotony and work dissatisfaction have also been implicated. Detailed assessment of individual factors can be complicated as several may be involved at the same time.

Several studies suggest an increased risk of low back pain in drivers of trucks, buses, tractors and in pilots. The more hours spent in a motor vehicle, the higher the risk of acute prolapsed intervertebral disc. Cigarette smoking in the previous year is also associated with an increased risk of prolapsed disc.[4]

Cervical and thoracic pain

People in the fourth decade of life are affected by a prolapsed cervical disc more than other age groups. Frequent lifting of heavy objects at work and cigarette smoking are clearly associated. Personal experience suggests that maintaining cervical flexion for prolonged periods (often seen in typists, computer operators, students and draughtsmen etc.) is a key factor. People who sleep prone (neck in rotation) or on their sides (if their neck is laterally flexed) may be predisposed to problems although there are no data to support this clinical impression. Some people give a clear history of pain arising after performing tasks with the neck in extension, e.g. painting ceilings.

MECHANICAL FACTORS

That mechanical factors are important in causing low back pain can be assumed by the recurrent histories of patients whose back was symptom-free until an abnormal strain was put on it. The mechanical load on the spine is increased by twisting movements against resistance, flexion of the spine and working with arms outstretched. There is a strong clinical impression that many episodes of back pain are initiated by bending from the waist with straight legs, and that these are far more common than episodes induced by heavy lifting. Extra strains are applied to the spine when, in flexion, there is added an additional movement such as twisting (rotation), or bending sideways (lateral flexion), or the strain of a cough or sneeze.

The effect of posture on the 'tension' of the spinal cord, roots and nerves is often neglected. Thus, sitting slumped forward with the head down and legs outstretched stresses all these structures, while in the cervical spine, symptoms of root irritation are often aggravated by carrying shopping. Similarly, the sciatic nerve may be stretched in certain postures, e.g. sitting, particularly in low easy chairs. Also of importance is the effect of various postures on intradiscal pressures.

ACUTE SPINAL PAIN

This discussion assumes difficulty in eliciting the precise anatomical origins of the pain, and outlines general principles of management which are of value irrespective of cause.

Where invasive techniques are not indicated, the options consist of general and physical measures, or drugs (Tables 2.1 and 2.2). Often rest and/ or support will be the mainstay. Frequently the positions adopted during rest are critical. Thus, for example, patients with a C5 lesion may work out for themselves how symptoms may be eased by placing their hand on top of their head. Conversely, patients advised to rest at home by their doctor because of acute sciatica often make their symptoms worse by spending their time sitting in a low chair.

General measures

These may largely consist of advice on pain-relieving positions (antalgic postures) and support (e.g. corset, soft collar, sling etc.).

Table 2.1   Therapeutic options in spinal pain

General measures
    Strict bed rest
    Local spinal support – collar, corset
    Avoidance of aggravating factors, e.g. standing still, sitting, bending and stooping,
    incorrect lifting, bad working postures
    Adjustment of lifestyle – e.g. avoid rushing about

Physical measures
    Mobilization techniques/manipulation/traction
    Manipulation under muscle relaxant or anaesthetic
    Exercises
    Postural training and self-care education
    Hydrotherapy
    Soft tissue techniques – massage
    Electrical treatments, e.g. interferential, ultrasound, pulsed short-wave diathermy
    Transcutaneous electrical nerve stimulation/acupuncture

Drugs – oral
    Pure analgesia
    Non-steroidal anti-inflammatory drugs
    Muscle relaxants, e.g. diazepam
    Tricyclic drugs, e.g. amitriptyline

Drugs – injection
    Local steroid injection with local anaesthetic, or by epidural route

Long-term measures
    Psychological assessment
    General toughening-up exercise programme
    Workshop assessment and treatment to assess:
        motivation and pain thresholds
        standing tolerance
        sitting tolerance
        time-keeping

Invasive measures – if indicated
    Chemonucleolysis
    Surgery

Antalgic postures

Pain, paraesthesiae and spasm may all be eased by taking physical stress off
irritable spinal structures. Suggestions for these can be made (Appendix 2.1)
but patients should be taught the general principles so they can intelligently
make their own modifications. Frequently, relief from one position is short-

Table 2.2   Illustrative flexible programme demonstrating some indications for physiotherapy in the acute stage

Relieve pain or paraesthesiae
Relieve muscle spasm
Increase range and quality of movement to improve function
Strengthen weak muscles
Improve posture and postural awareness during various activities
Analyse patients' work/leisure situations
Assist in motivation
Restore confidence and encourage earliest feasible return to work/activities

lived and another needs to be substituted. In an attempt to relieve pain, many patients develop poor postures which may persist as a bad habit, creating problems for the future, and thus they require advice even at this early stage.

Physical measures

Additional symptom relief may be obtained from physiotherapy arranged from a hospital clinic, although many district general hospitals now operate an 'open access' scheme to enable general practitioners to refer such patients directly. The patient is assessed by a chartered physiotherapist who selects the most appropriate form of treatment aimed at the earliest restoration of range and function. This might include a form of passive segmental mobilization (Maitland techniques), teaching the patient specific methods of exercises (e.g. McKenzie passive extensions[5]), using adjunct pain-relieving techniques (see Table 2.1) or supplying a support. If trauma has resulted in much soft tissue involvement (e.g. some fractures, whiplash injury) electrical treatment such as pulsed shortwave, interferential or ultrasound may be used. From the earliest stages of treatment, advice is given on posture and spinal care, and an analysis of spinal use over the 24-hour period is performed so patients learn how to avoid aggravating symptoms both at work and at leisure (see section on posture training and education, below).

Drug management

Drug treatment may be important in the management of acute spinal pain. Three classes of drugs will be considered: non-steroidal anti-inflammatory drugs (NSAIDs), simple analgesics, and muscle relaxants. NSAIDs are invaluable in management as they perform two separate functions: they are undoubtedly effective analgesics, and a group of them have a 12-hour duration of action for which there is no pure analgesic substitute. This is important as NSAIDs taken as tablets or suppositories late in the evening can have an analgesic effect during the night and ease the stiffness and pain which are so often found to be worse on waking in the morning. In addition, they may prevent people from waking in the middle of the night when they turn in bed; this may be exquisitely painful for patients with acute spinal conditions. It is likely, however, that they also play a role as anti-inflammatory agents, possibly reducing the inflammatory response around disc, joint, or soft tissues, any of which may be the cause of the patient's pain. The choice of agent will depend on the severity of the pain and the possible risk of side-effects. Clearly, prescribing drugs that make people vomit will not improve their spinal pain. Where patients have a history of gastrointestinal upset in the past, if simple analgesics are inadequate, the addition of ranitidine or cimetidine to the drug regimen may allow the NSAID to be tolerated.

Pure analgesics may be given without risk of mucosal damage to the gastrointestinal tract but again potency and side-effects tend to be linked. Paracetamol may be effective in the elderly but is seldom helpful in the younger patient with acute severe spinal pain. The compound paracetamol-containing analgesic drugs (with codeine, dihydrocodeine, or dextropropoxyphene) are sometimes needed. Both codeine and dihydrocodeine may give rise to nausea or vomiting, and aggravate the constipation consequent upon bed rest. For patients in very severe pain, buprenorphine, meptazinol, or nefopam may all be worth trying. Opiates are only very seldom necessary for a limited period.

Muscle relaxants have been prescribed for many years but are rarely used in our practice. Occasionally diazepam is helpful as it has additional sedative properties, which may benefit a small group of patients. Diazepam used in this situation should be given for short periods only in view of the increasingly recognized problems that may follow the establishment of diazepam dependence.

ACUTE PAIN ARISING FROM THE NECK AND THORAX

Trauma is a major cause of acute cervical pain, and whiplash injuries from road traffic accidents are common. People may wake up with severe cervical pain. The pain may be localized to the neck, or referred to the head, face, shoulder girdle, chest and/or upper limbs. Paraesthesiae or numbness may be associated.

Acute severe chest pain may be referred from the cervical or thoracic spine and is often confused with cardiac pain. It may be the cause of unnecessary referrals to the Accident & Emergency Department in the middle of the night. The pain is usually but not always unilateral, superficial, and often associated with tenderness over the pectoral muscles, ribs, or costochondral junctions. Management consists of postural advice, physiotherapy (see below), and NSAIDs.

Acute abdominal pain referred from the spine is usually a diagnosis of exclusion, although a careful history of pain radiating to or from the spine may be obtained, or pain may be reproduced by rotation of the spine.

Management

Immediate provision of a soft collar (and/or a sling) is often appropriate where acute pain arises from the neck or cervicodorsal junction. Assuming a degree of oedema around cervical structures, NSAIDs (see above) appear logical. Bed rest is seldom needed; most people remain mobile with the aid of a support. If pain is very severe rest with appropriate positioning of the spine and limbs (see Appendix 2.1), analgesia, and possibly a sedative type of muscle relaxant, e.g. diazepam, may be required for a few days.

Collars

To fulfil its function, a collar should fit snugly under the jaw and head above and rest on the clavicles and adjacent soft tissues below, thus partly helping to take the weight of the head. 'Instant' collars are available but unless they coincide with the patient's measurements, or can be altered to do so, they are of no use. Indeed, a collar that pushes the head or neck into an inappropriate position may well aggravate symptoms. Made to measure soft collars can usually be obtained from the physiotherapy department at the local hospital as part of an immediate programme but some practitioners may prefer to make their own. Instructions for making one type of soft collar are given in Appendix 2.2. When there are no facilities for making a soft collar, a towel folded several times, wound round the neck and secured with a tie, or a folded newspaper padded with a scarf may be of value.

Initially it is possible for dexterity and/or co-ordination to be impaired while wearing the collar, and patients should also be warned against moving around in complete darkness while wearing one, as they may overbalance. A collar should be withdrawn as soon as possible to avoid dependence, but where it has been worn by day as well as at night, it is usually best to have a

Table 2.3 Suggested indications for a collar

Acute cervical pain and spasm

Pain worse in morning, particularly for restless sleepers (soft collar only)

Occipital and other symptoms arising from the neck

Pain on neck movements, not controlled by other measures

weaning off period, rather than instant removal. A patient should also be advised to keep the collar (stored flat if a soft one) in case of future need.

Fusion/rigid collars are relatively rarely required, their main indication being in cases either of vertebro-basilar insufficiency or instability, when patients may be unsuitable for, or awaiting, surgery.

At the best of times, these collars are not comfortable to wear so it is vitally important that they are skilfully tailored for the individual by an expert with access to a range of suitable materials. Some indications for using a collar are listed in Table 2.3.

Slings

When symptoms in the arm are severe and aggravated by any downward drag of the limb, a webbing sling can take the weight off the arm, thus easing pain, paraesthesiae and spasm, without placing undue strain on the neck (see Fig. 2.2). This may be obtained from hospital or can easily be homemade. An average size requires 1.5 metres of 5-cm wide furniture webbing obtainable from upholsterers and some hardware or carpet stores. Loops to support the patient's forearm below the elbow and at the wrist may be stitched or stapled in place, but a nappy pin has the advantage of enabling the sling to be lengthened for use over a coat. As with other supports, it should be dispensed with as soon as it is no longer required.

Physical measures

Physical measures are as for acute spinal pain (see p. 48).

ACUTE LOW BACK PAIN

Although acute low back pain develops insidiously in some, or is noted on waking in others, many episodes have a clearly defined cause. Acute trauma

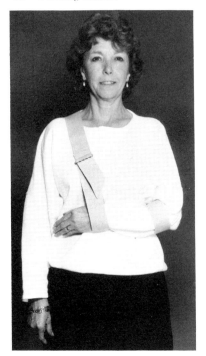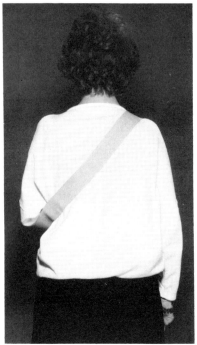

Fig. 2.2   Illustration of a webbing sling used to reduce any aggravation of pain, paraesthesiae or spasm in the neck by downward drag of an arm

or incident (e.g. bending with straight legs to put an article into a cupboard) usually gives immediate pain, which may gradually worsen during the day, and will often be at its most severe on waking next morning. Where an accident or injury has taken place more than 48 hours before the onset of any symptoms, experience suggests there is unlikely to be a causal relationship. Severe episodes of low back pain may well develop sciatica after a period of up to 2 weeks.

Management

The role of physiotherapy in the management of acute low back pain varies, as some physicians and therapists are more likely to favour early intervention than others. Some studies suggest that early physiotherapy may decrease symptoms more rapidly than rest where physiotherapy is available to general practitioners. The principles of physiotherapy have been outlined above

(p. 48). The alternative management is rest in the appropriate position, analgesia, NSAIDs and the avoidance of aggravating factors.

Bed rest at home

Many people find bed rest satisfactory, and the importance of bedding is emphasized below. Some prefer resting in the main room of the house (possibly with a mattress on the floor), where television may help ease the monotony, and heating may be conserved. Often the close proximity of a toilet will dictate where rest takes place. Those with severe pain aggravated by weight-bearing when walking may be helped by the provision of elbow crutches by the domiciliary physiotherapy service. The community nursing service may provide a commode by the bed. Bed rest at home beyond 3 weeks is seldom indicated for mechanical back pain. Intractable pain beyond this period is an indication for specialist advice, as inappropriate prolonged rest increases physical debility and psychological dependence.

Mobilization following bed rest should be gradual. Patients should be advised to avoid any form of lifting or bending. Sitting for longer than 5–10 minutes may aggravate symptoms, particularly if sciatica is present. Gentle walking can alternate with resting in the appropriate posture (Appendix 2.1). The patient must wait until the next morning to ensure no aggravation of pain has occurred from the previous day's activities. It is important to try to avoid constipation as straining at stool may aggravate spinal symptoms. For this reason, codeine derivatives are best avoided if possible, and the community nursing service may be involved.

The elderly patient should have minimal bed rest to prevent excessive stiffness in the short term and demineralization of bone in the long term. Early mobilization may be facilitated by a temporary corset fitted as soon as the patient is well enough to go to hospital. Occasionally the surgical fitter may be available to make a domiciliary visit.

Lumbar supports

There is no good evidence to support the use of corsets, but many clinicians find them of great value. Their mode of action is unclear, though a well-fitting support will increase the intra-abdominal pressure. They undoubtedly help in restoring confidence for some patients, and facilitate mobilization after an acute episode of back pain for others. They may encourage a better posture in some patients. The most useful support is a temporary one, fitted immediately, and if it is to be of value it should be comfortable during sitting. Custom-made corsets may take some weeks to

Table 2.4   Suggested indications for corset

Mobilization following bed rest after acute back pain

Mechanical instability, e.g. spondylolisthesis

Back pain aggravated by spinal movements inadequately controlled by physiotherapy, posture, drugs etc.

For support during heavy activities, such as gardening, heavy work etc.

---

produce, but any corset must be checked by the prescriber to ensure a satisfactory fit, and that the patient understands how to put it on, and is willing to wear it. Unless the patient is on income support, a charge will be made under the NHS, currently £14.00 (subject to change). Many patients find the belt tends to slip upwards, in spite of the stabilizing strap. In women this may be helped by wearing a pantie-girdle over the belt. For some men, a wide leather or canvas belt, as worn by weight lifters, may work well as a corset substitute.

The prescription of a corset should be linked with the performance of regular exercises aimed at preventing loss of muscle tone.

Suggested indications for use of a corset are listed in Table 2.4 and when symptoms are controlled, a 'weaning out of the corset' process may be attempted over some weeks. Some people continue to wear supports just for at-risk activities, such as gardening. As with collars, patients are advised not to discard their corset – it may be useful for another episode of low back pain.

RELAPSING AND CHRONIC SPINAL PAIN

Many people with spinal pain become pain-free after a period but may be liable to relapses. A small proportion may have persisting pain over months or years. The profusion of treatments available (Table 2.1) suggests the extent of our ignorance about management. At this stage, the symptoms are usually more of persistent, nagging discomfort, which may arise from:

1. The continual stress of faulty posture at work or leisure on otherwise normal structures.
2. The poorly resolved aftermath of an acute episode (e.g. whiplash, acute disc).
3. Stresses on already chronically degenerated structures.

Table 2.5 Illustrative flexible physiotherapy programme for chronic spinal pain

Symptom control – pain and paraesthesiae

Improving range and quality of movement:
    mobilizing joint structures
    stretching tight tissues
    improving stability and strength

Improvement of static and dynamic postures

Analysis of work and leisure postures and movements over 24 hours

Encouraging patient self-criticism of activities to avoid aggravation of symptoms

Supporting and motivating patient and family through the psychological consequences of pain and disability

Facilitating optimal return to previous work and leisure activities

Advising on alternative employment or retraining – referral to disablement resettlement officer

Management

The key to management is to train people how to select those postures and methods of using the body that minimize stresses and do not aggravate symptoms, thus helping to reduce the likelihood of recurrence. For advice of this kind, together with other physical measures that could be of benefit, the patient can be referred to a physiotherapy department. A coinciding course of drug therapy (see below) should also be considered.

Physical measures

Aims of treatment are listed in Tables 2.5 and 2.6. Methods would probably involve passive mobilizing/manipulative techniques to loosen stiffened

Table 2.6 Rationale for exercise

To mobilize stiff areas of the spine generally and/or segmentally

To stabilize locally and/or regionally

To redress imbalance by specific strengthening

To stretch shortened or adherent structures

To improve posture and postural awareness

To retrain forgotten 'normal' patterns of movement

structures and stretch tight or adherent tissues (e.g. sciatic nerve). This would be reinforced by teaching the patient methods of doing these exercises at home. Exercise regimens to improve strength or stability may be necessary and other techniques may prove useful adjuncts (see Table 2.1). A full programme of self-care education should also be included as a preventive measure (see section on posture training and education, p. 61).

If an 'open access' scheme is in operation accepting this type of patient, a general practitioner may refer the patient directly for treatment; otherwise it is necessary for a consultant to do this. All options listed would probably be available from a good rehabilitation department in a district general hospital. Chartered physiotherapists are trained to examine and assess for suitable techniques those patients for whom physiotherapy is likely to be beneficial and to recognize when or if these are not succeeding and should be discontinued. Since 1977 (see DHSS Health Circular HC (77) 33), chartered physiotherapists have been held responsible for any therapy they administer. Thus it is not good practice to prescribe specific techniques, nor to promise the patient a particular form of treatment (e.g. heat) which the therapist may feel inappropriate. Descriptions of specific techniques of treatment are outside the scope of this chapter. The rationale of exercise is listed in Table 2.6. Exercise schemes vary according to need and operator.

If patients have had a prolonged period of bed rest prior to referral, resulting in lack of confidence or marked stiffness, hydrotherapy may be useful, and is often also of great value after surgery.

Transcutaneous electrical nerve stimulation (TENS) is now widely used to attempt to control pain for which other measures were unsuccessful and when surgery is not contemplated. If successful, TENS may be continued indefinitely at home, with patients having their own machine. Patients may be admitted to hospital for assessment, when the optimum site for placement of electrodes, pulse frequency and duration of treatment are decided. Some centres assess people as outpatients, and may loan stimulators from the pain clinic or the physiotherapy department. In other districts patients are requested to purchase their own equipment (see Fig. 1.1).

Acupuncture is now frequently offered by pain clinics and some physiotherapy departments. Currently it is not possible to predict which patients will do well with either TENS or acupuncture.

Drug management

The principles of drug management have been outlined above (pp. 48–9). Analgesia is usually best achieved with NSAIDs but many patients referred for a second opinion have not had this form of treatment. Achieving freedom from night pain is very important. A good night's rest can make daytime pain tolerable. Sometimes NSAIDs are a necessary adjunct to physiotherapy, with the two measures having a synergistic effect. Intermittent analgesia is sensible, and patients must feel that they have an effective analgesic available when their pain is overwhelming. This is explored in greater depth on pp. 13–15.

There is no role for muscle relaxants at this stage, and virtually none for tranquilizers. Patients who are anxious and have difficulty in sleeping, or in whom social or emotional factors are playing a part in perpetuating their pain, may require tricyclic antidepressants (see section on drug treatment, below).

Chronic cervical pain

This problem is so common that it warrants a separate mention. In practice, it is very rare for there to be a sinister underlying cause for chronic neck pain. The general, physical and drug management is identical to that described above. It is helpful, however, for patients to treat their spine as if they had low back pain; avoid sleeping on sagging mattresses and always maintain a good posture, whether standing or sitting, at work or at leisure.

Whilst good neck posture may follow from a good overall back posture, sufferers from neck pain should always modify tasks which need cervical extension, e.g. looking upwards to paint a ceiling. Prolonged leaning forwards is best avoided. Changes of posture every 15–20 minutes (particularly getting up from sitting) are recommended.

Advice on lying and sitting posture (see section on posture training and education, p. 61; Fig. 2.3 and Appendix 2.1) is critical. Occasionally pain relief is not obtained after following advice, physiotherapy and medication. A firm collar is then worth considering (see section on collars, pp. 50–1).

THE 'DIFFICULT' BACK PAIN

Whilst most episodes of spinal pain are self-limiting, for reasons that are unclear some patients have persisting disabling pain in spite of many of the measures that have been mentioned above. These have usually included NSAIDs, analgesics, and physiotherapy, and may also have included treatment from heterodox practitioners. Investigations (often including radiculography) have usually been performed without positive results. These people may have pain from any part of the spine, but classically suffer from low back pain.

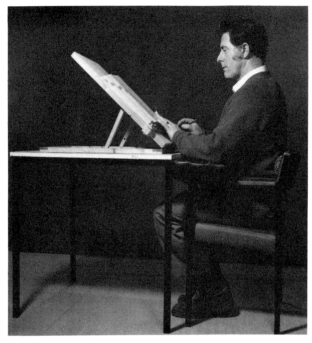

Fig. 2.3   Illustration of the use of a lumbar roll to support the back, use of an arm rest to decrease downward drag of the arm and use of an easel to inhibit neck flexion

It has to be determined whether physical or psychological factors are most likely to be influencing current symptoms. Often both will coexist, but on occasions it will be clear that either the physical or the psychological is predominating. Although for the sake of clarity they are described separately, the two aspects of management must go hand in hand.

Physical aspects of management

A clue that physical aspects remain important may lie in the pattern of pain. If the pain is episodic and related to movement or posture, physical causes are likely to predominate. Often continual faulty posture at work or leisure places abnormal stress on normal tissue, or causes recurrent stress on chronically degenerate structures. Management consists of helping the sufferer to understand how mechanical factors may be aggravating the pain, and how such mechanical stresses may be lessened or avoided.

Another important area to question is that of sleep. After checking that the bedding and mattress are satisfactory (see section on bedding and mattresses, pp. 63–65), it is important to ascertain whether the loss of sleep is due to pain, insomnia or depression. If pain is constant, both day and night, then depression or psychosocial factors need to be evaluated. The pain which wakes the patient purely when he or she is turning over in sleep may be helped with NSAIDs. On occasions, questioning what is thought about when lying awake gives a clue to social factors which may reflect the causes or the consequences of the spinal condition.

A minority of spinal patients, usually with low back pain, may be 'off sick' for prolonged periods, and have difficulty in returning to work. Problems arise from the fear that employment may aggravate their pain, or cause it to recur; the prolonged adoption of the patient role, which may discourage a positive approach to work; the loss of self-discipline which may result in poor time-keeping; and the lack of stamina and strength due to prolonged inactivity, which may have been consequent to bed rest. Such people can be helped by a general 'toughening-up' in the physiotherapy department, and/ or supervision of a gradually increasing range of activities in the occupational therapy department. These activities may require working through pain to develop stamina and the ability to cope with sitting, standing and lifting. The exercises can be increased to mimic a full day at work. This reassures both patient and staff that such a course is likely to be successful.[6]

This type of rehabilitation programme should be available at any district general hospital, and is suitable for outpatients. When outpatient rehabilitation fails, or if it is not available locally, patients should be offered a residential assessment in the rehabilitation ward of the district general hospital, or at a medical rehabilitation unit. Here a thorough medical, nursing, psychological, remedial therapeutic and social assessment can take place as the patient is under observation for the whole of the 24-hour period.

Psychological and social aspects of management

A significant group of patients present with pain which is continuous and which apparently does not alter over the 24-hour period. They are best considered as suffering from the 'pain behaviour syndrome'. Examination may not reveal physical signs compatible with the disability described consequent upon the pain. The pattern of pain referral may be 'non-anatomical'.[7] Examination, particularly of the straight leg raise test, is accompanied by exaggerated gestures of pain.[7,8] Insomnia is frequent and worthy of examination (see above). Patients may admit to problems consequent upon loss of earnings, or upon changing marital relationships. Experienced doctors and therapists often uncover unrealistic fears, e.g. that long-standing pain cannot be due to common musculoskeletal causes, and must be caused by cancer or multiple sclerosis. The fear of aggravating the pain may act as an excessive inhibition, keeping patients inactive and away from work unnecessarily. The effect on the spouse may be critical, particularly if over-protection or excessive sympathy has encouraged an individual to adopt a patient role.

As in other disabling conditions, prolonged back pain, particularly if it results in time off work, may put a strain on marital and family relationships by virtue of the partners being in more continual close contact with each other, and one being unable to fulfil the normal obligations to the other. Thus a heavy manual worker unable to continue work may find dependence on the spouse for earnings an unbearable strain. This subject is explored in greater detail in Chapter 5 (on stroke). Where the marital relationship has been difficult prior to the onset of back pain, the pain may be used as an excuse to withdraw from the sexual side of the partnership, putting further strain upon the relationship. Not all patients will be able to continue a normal sexual relationship when in severe pain, but many people can be helped by the intelligent use of positioning.

Compensation may be another complicating problem. Once medical reports have been obtained from both parties, patients can be assured that the basis for a settlement is highly likely and that they must now concentrate on positive matters, e.g. a return to work, the development of new interests, looking after the family whilst the spouse works etc.

It may take a long time to unravel the many psychological and social problems that have become associated with an individual's pain. Not all problems can be resolved, but the time taken to come to grips with them is often therapeutic and may enable back pain sufferers and their families to cope with life again. Sometimes specialist counselling is required from a social worker or a psychologist. The latter is also helpful in advising the rehabilitation team on possible behavioural approaches to management. Usually both physical and behavioural managements are combined simultaneously, with the presence of therapists often being essential to give the individual an 'excuse' to get better.

Drug treatment

Investigations in this group of patients will have excluded treatable causes of nociceptive pain and the rationale of simple analgesics and NSAIDs is therefore reduced. Many patients at this stage may be taking a number of drugs, including simple analgesics, and careful enquiry as to the effectiveness of each drug must be made; when in doubt it should be stopped.

Where patients do admit to marked variations in pain related to posture or activity, mechanical explanations continue to be likely, and if NSAIDs have not been tried they should be, particularly if sleep is disturbed by pain. When one of the 12-hourly duration of action NSAIDs is appropriate (see pp. 48–9) but ineffective, and where mechanical factors are still thought to be playing a major role, stronger analgesics such as nefopam, meptazinol or buprenorphine may be worth a trial, but should be discontinued rapidly if there is no dramatic effect. Caution needs to be taken with the more powerful analgesic drugs in old age, where side-effects arising from the central nervous system such as dizziness, sedation, or confusion may result.

Patients not responding to analgesics or NSAIDs may be helped by tricyclic antidepressant drugs, and these are often beneficial even in the absence of depression. The mode of action is not entirely clear. The tricyclic compounds with sedative side-effects such as amitriptyline or nortriptyline may be helpful, as the sedation can be used to facilitate sleep. In this situation the precise timing of the taking of tablets can best be adjusted by the individual to minimize unwanted sedation in the evening, and the hangover effect in the morning. Thus many patients may take amitriptyline at about 18.00 h. They need to be warned of the sedative side-effects and also the dry mouth. Patients in this group need to be specifically advised that the tablets are being taken to help their chronic pain, and are not being prescribed as antidepressants, as patients are often non-compliant if they think they are being treated for depression.

Employment

When a rehabilitation programme clarifies the fact that patients will not be able to return to their previous work, referral to the disablement resettlement officer (DRO) may be helpful. The DRO can discuss with employers alternative work which should be within the clients' capabilities, register people as 'disabled' and help them to find work in a variety of ways. Where no such work is available, advice is given about other job options or retirement on the grounds of ill health.

Younger people (under 40–45) may be referred to an employment rehabilitation centre (ERC) where they are assessed for their retraining potential.

POSTURE TRAINING AND EDUCATION

All patients referred for physiotherapy should be offered advice on posture and reorganization of the environments encountered by them over a 24-hour period. Experience has shown, however, that often education gets squeezed out of the timetable of a hard-pressed doctor or physiotherapist. Thus many hospitals have developed a group back education programme to reinforce the understanding by patients of the underlying nature of back problems. The importance of self-help in limiting current symptoms and the prevention of recurrence are stressed.

Unlike the original 'back schools' of the USA and Scandinavia, some British programmes are designed for all back pain sufferers, not just the very severely disabled ones. One such programme is outlined in Table 2.7. This approach has the advantage of bringing patients together (Fig. 2.4) so that they can appreciate that their problems are shared by many others, and mutual support can be given. These programmes are usually cost-effective. Inevitably in the group situation an over-simplified view is offered, and patients should be given enough insight to modify the advice to suit their individual needs. All patients are helped to understand the responsibility they have for themselves and this may be reinforced by the use of leaflets which act as a permanent reminder.

The following points are emphasized:

1. The maintenance of well balanced static and dynamic postures.
2. Simple reorganization of work methods, e.g. frequent changes of position or task.
3. Simple reorganization of working surfaces by slanting (e.g. the use of desk easels for reading/writing; see Fig. 2.3), raising or lowering; the placement of visual displays just below the horizontal.
4. The avoidance of particular postures, usually with the spine in flexion or

Table 2.7   A back education programme in four sessions

Session 1	Demonstration of spinal anatomy (Fig. 2.4), mechanics, ergonomics, correct postural habits and lifting techniques – making use of visual aids, etc.
Session 2	Demonstration of the management of daily activities by an occupational therapist in the patient's living area or workshop
Session 3	Teaching individualized exercise programme – reinforcement of postural advice and lifting techniques
Session 4	Open forum – questions and answers – checking and modifications of exercise regimens. Opportunity for group feedback
	When hydrotherapy is available, a couple of sessions may be added to encourage exercise and fitness through swimming

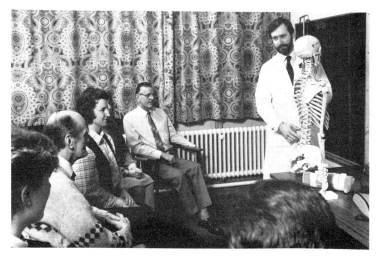

Fig. 2.4 Demonstration of spinal anatomy in the Northwick Park Hospital Back Education Programme

extension, where cervical pathology may cause giddiness (e.g. looking up whilst climbing a ladder).
5. Good lifting and handling techniques.
6. The importance of keeping the spine mobile by putting it through a full range of movement, especially stretching, which should include the anterior muscles of the thorax and shoulder girdle.
7. The importance of keeping generally fit – swimming is usually recommended for confident swimmers with spinal problems.

Samples of some of the hints offered are given in Tables 2.8 and 2.9.

Patients attending this type of back education programme are usually in one of two categories. For some the course is the only stage necessary in their treatment (particularly suitable for those who have recovered from an attack of low back pain and are currently symptom-free). For others it represents the final stage, following previous treatment, e.g. physiotherapy or surgery.

BEDDING AND MATTRESSES

The texture of mattress and pillow is important. Some people with low back pain find very firm or orthopaedic mattresses helpful, but tend to be a minority of sufferers. Often such people have found relief by lying supine on

Table 2.8   Some suggestions for people with spinal pain

Things to avoid

Prolonged leaning forward, e.g. by use of long-handled garden tools; bath/change nappy/dress baby on high table with everything handy

Non-stop driving (longer than 30 minutes)

Soft or unyielding mattress

Low easy chairs

Lifting with a bent spine or with outstretched arms

Jerking or twisting the spine

Overstretching, e.g. reaching into high cupboards

Uneven loading of spine, e.g. shopping should be carried in two evenly weighted bags

Things to consider

Frequent changes in posture during routine activities

Seating modifications at work (Fig. 2.3.)

Use small lumbar supports in seats (Fig. 2.3.)

Use castors on heavy furniture, e.g. fridge

Use webbings to assist lifting awkward furniture, e.g. wardrobe (See Figs. 2.5–2.6)

Regular exercise, e.g. swimming

Sweep and brush with a sideways action from upright posture

---

the floor, or on a mattress on the floor. Others, by contrast, have found their pain aggravated by very hard mattresses. The majority, in our experience, are helped by firm but not unyielding mattresses, which have some superficial 'give', thus enabling the mattress to contour to the shape of the patient's spine. For those with sagging mattresses, a board placed underneath is a useful temporary measure. Some people will wish to purchase more appropriate bedding. When buying a mattress they should be advised to lie on it in various positions for at least a quarter of an hour. Many have found the extra expense of pocket-sprung mattresses worthwhile.

Pillows are best made of down. Feather pillows may be satisfactory, but solid foam pillows are contraindicated as they cannot be shaped.

Symptoms can be aggravated by the simple task of getting into or out of bed, and arranging the bed so that it is at a convenient height is a prerequisite of management. Most beds are too low and may be raised by bed blocks

Table 2.9 Hints to avoid bending and stooping

Task	Method
Washing up	Raise bowel within sink or use high stool to sit on*
Ironing	Use adjustable-height ironing board Use high stool*
Loading washing machine or dish washer	Kneel to load. Use front loaders For top-loading washing machines use tongs
Making beds	Perform kneeling – consider duvets
Cleaning bath	Clean from inside Kneel outside Use short-handled mop and rinse with shower attachment
Brushing teeth	Do sitting*
Washing hair	Stand upright using shower attachment
Picking up	From kneeling or squatting position Use 'helping hand' for light objects if unable to kneel, e.g. osteoarthritic knees (Fig. 1.6)
For older people Getting up	High chairs High toilet seats Appropriate height of bed

*Sometimes sitting to avoid standing can be counterproductive. Some people find 'lodging' on the edge of a high stool a useful substitute (Fig. 2.7).

of equal size under all legs of the bed. For people who suffer from hiatus hernia, ischaemic heart disease, left ventricular failure, and even anxiety when lying flat, raising the head of the bed with blocks may be helpful.

Duvets may be more comfortable than heavy blankets, and have the great advantage of minimizing bed-making!

SEATING

Many people spend large proportions of their day sitting down and the postures adopted then may have a direct influence on their spinal pain. Three important areas relate to sitting – work, home, and when travelling. The important principles to consider are the height of the seat from the ground, and the depth of the squab (seat of the chair). These will vary from one indi-

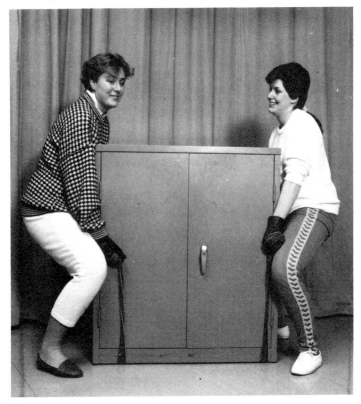

Fig. 2.5a   Use of webbing to assist in lifting bulky objects

vidual to another – ideally the feet should rest comfortably on the floor with the knees at approximately 90°, and with 5–7 cm leeway between the front of the squab and the back of the knee. This allows free movement of the legs and facilitates standing up from the chair. Seats may be raised with extra cushions or firmed by placing a board under the cushion and resting on the chair frame. Usually the chair which supports the lumbar lordos gives most comfort. Portable inflatable supports may be bought and have the advantage of being variable in the degree of inflation, thus allowing a change in spinal position.

Arm rests at an appropriate height are often useful because they prevent drooping of the shoulder girdle. Many chairs, however, have low arm rests which encourage slouching. Such chairs can easily be modified with cushions or foam blocks on the arms (see Fig. 2.3).

Elderly people who may also have peripheral arthritis require chairs that

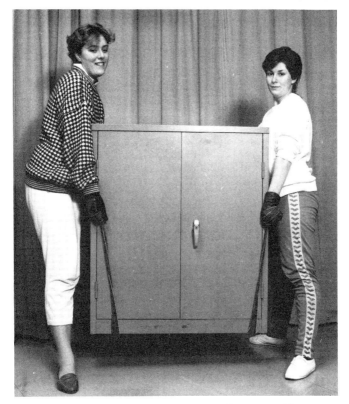

Fig. 2.5b Use of webbing to assist in lifting bulky objects

are high off the ground, have high straight backs, and arm rests that facilitate getting in and out of the chair (see p. 29).

More recently, seating of a Scandinavian design which encourages maintenance of the lumbar lordos has become available in the UK. The seat pitches forwards and anterior tibial supports stabilize the position (Fig. 2.8). For those who find this comfortable, Granny's rocking chair can be modified to advantage (Fig. 2.9). A foam wedge on the seat of a conventional chair promoting a slightly forward pitch may also be comfortable and encourage a good posture whilst allowing the legs to move freely.

We believe many chairs in use for people with predominantly sedentary occupations are unsatisfactory from the viewpoint of supporting the spine. The commonest problems are that the height of the seat is inappropriate to the height of the work surface, encouraging a bad posture, and back support, where present, is often badly positioned.

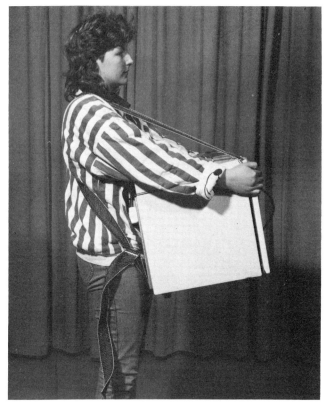

Fig. 2.6   Use of webbing to assist in lifting bulky objects

THE CAR

A car may be essential to maintain an independent life and many people require it to earn their living, get to work, take children to school, and to do the shopping. The following points are worth considering.

Whiplash injuries can be minimized by the use of head restraints of sufficient height and proximity so that the occiput can be supported. A common misconception is that restraints should only go to the level of the neck and this can in fact aggravate a whiplash injury.

For people with low back pain there is no ideal seat. The more variations in seat position there are on a model, the more likely the individual is to be suited. An adjustable slope of the back rest may be valuable, particularly for those who prefer their seat to be more upright. Some support for the lumbar

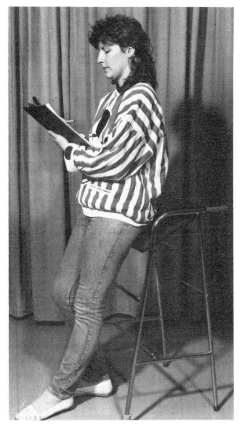

Fig. 2.7 Painful prolonged standing may be ameliorated by lodging on the edge of a high stool

curve is essential and lateral supports for trunk and thighs are helpful. A variety of back rests and seating wedges for use in car seats are available, with many costing less than £20. If back rests do not provide the answer, and the individual does not want to replace the car, replacement car seats are available. Some have an adjustable squab (cushion of seat) length and this is advantageous for tall drivers. Seats are available costing from £50 to £300.

Mothers with young children are advised to use four-door rather than two-door cars in order to minimize bending and stretching when strapping children into rear seats.

For those using their cars to carry goods regularly, whether the goods are bags of groceries, or promotional material for representatives, consideration

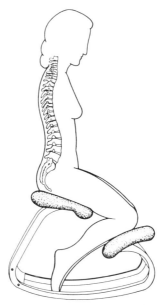

Fig. 2.8 Scandinavian design chair demonstrating maintenance of the lumbar lordos

should be given to purchasing either an estate or a hatchback car which has a boot with a level surface. People using the boot can then squat or kneel and slide things in and out of the car without having to lift over a ledge.

As in other aspects of living with spinal pain, frequent changes of posture are recommended, and we suggest people stop driving after 20 to 30 minutes in order to get out of the car, have a stretch and a stroll for 1 or 2 minutes, and then continue on their way. People should be advised to leave plenty of time for their journey so that they are not driving under stress and have time for such stops.

THE VOLUNTARY SECTOR

The addresses of the Back Pain Society, and the Back Pain Research Society are given in Chapter 14.

The Arthritis and Rheumatism Council produces a number of leaflets about rheumatic conditions (see Chapter 1, Appendix 1.1), and those on neck pain, backache and seating are well worth recommending to appropriate patients with spinal pain.

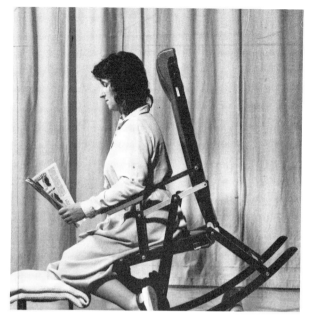

Fig. 2.9 Use of a rocking chair to encourage maintenance of the lumbar lordos

CONCLUSIONS

Spinal pain is extremely common, usually mild, but sometimes may be very distressing. A strong emphasis on self-care is inherent in management, and if skilled advice is available early, loss of morale following prolonged pain is often avoided. The commonest aggravating factors involve bending the spine inappropriately, often with coincidental lifting, twisting or other repetitive postures, and these habits can often be corrected with marked improvement of symptoms. For the minority of patients with severe or long-standing idiopathic low back pain, a careful understanding of the social and psychological factors which may be partly associated with cause, or with the consequences of the pain, may assist in management. Drugs may help at all stages of management.

REFERENCES

1. Wells N. (1985), *Back Pain*, London, Office of Health Economics.

2. Jayson M. I. V. (1984), Difficult diagnoses in back pain, *Br. Med. J.*; **288**: 741–2.
3. Waddell G. (1982), An approach to backache, *Br. J. Hosp. Med.*; **28**: 187–219.
4. Kelsey J. L., Gittens P. B., O'Connor T. et al (1984), Acute prolapsed interverte-bral disc – an epidemiological study with special reference to driving automobiles and to cigarette smoking, *Spine*; **9**: 608–13.
5. McKenzie R. A. (1981), *The Lumbar Spine – Mechanical Diagnosis and Therapy*, Waikanae, New Zealand, Spinal Publications.
6. Frank A. O., Henshaw D. J., Parkin D. R. (1987), Industrial therapy for physical disability in a district hospital rehabilitation unit, *Care, Sci. Pract.*; **5**: 29–33.
7. Ransford A. O., Cairns D., Mooney V. (1976), The pain drawing as an aid to the evaluation of patients with low back pain, *Spine*; **1**: 127–34.
8. Waddell G., McCullough J. A., Kummel E., Venner R. M. (1980), Nonorganic physical signs in low back pain. *Spine*; **5**: 117–25.

FURTHER READING

Bulstrode S. J., Harrison R. A., Clark A. K. (1983), *Assessments of Back Rests for Use in Car Seats. DHSS Aids Assessment Programme*, London, HMSO.

Bulstrode S. J., Harrison R. A., Clark A. K. (1985), *Assessment of Replacement Car Seats. DHSS Aids Assessment Programme*, London, HMSO.

Coxhead C. E., Meade T. W., Inskip H., North W. R. S., Troup J. D. G. (1981), Multicentre trial of physiotherapy in the management of sciatic symptoms, *Lancet*; **1**: 1065–8.

DHSS (1979), *Working Group on Back Pain: Report to Secretary of State for Social Services* (Chairman: Prof. A. L. Cochrane), London, HMSO.

Glossop E. S., Williams I. M. (1982), Increased patient compliance with exercises by use of booklets, *Demonstration Centres in Rehabilitation Newsletter*; **28**: 41–50.

Grieve G. P. (1981), *Common Vertebral Joint Problems* Edinburgh, Churchill Living-stone.

Grieve G. P. ed. (1986), *Modern Manual Therapy of the Vertebral Column*, London, Churchill Livingstone.

Harris G., Kendall R., Williams I., Frank A. O. (1982), Northwick Park Hospital Back Education Programme, *Demonstration Centres in Rehabilitation Newsletter:* **28**: 62–3.

Jayson M. I. V., Sims-Williams H., Young S. et al (1981), Mobilisation and manip-ulation for low back pain, *Spine*; **6**: 409–16.

Klaber Moffett J. A., Chase S. M., Portek I., Ennis J. R. (1986), A controlled, pro-spective study to evaluate the effectiveness of a back school in the relief of chronic low back pain, *Spine*; **11**: 120–2.

Maitland G. D. (1986), *Vertebral Manipulation*, 5th edn, London, Butterworths.

McKenzie A. (1980), *Treat Your Own Back*, Waikanae, New Zealand, Spinal Publi-cations.

McKenzie R. A. (1983), *Treat Your Own Neck*, Waikanae, New Zealand, Spinal Publications.

Nachemson A., Morris J. M. (1964), In vivo measurement of intradiscal pressure, *J. Bone Joint Surg.*; **46A**: 1077–92.

Scott J. T., ed. (1986), *Copeman's Textbook of the Rheumatic Diseases*, London, Churchill Livingstone.

Stoddard A. (1979), *The Back – Relief from Pain*, London, Martin Dunitz.

Wells P., Frampton V., Bowsher D. (1988), *Pain: Management and control in physio-therapy*, London, Heinemann Medical Books.

Wood P. H. N., Badley E. M. (1980), Epidemiology of back pain, in *The Lumbar Spine and Back Pain*, 2nd edn, (Jayson M.I.V., ed.) Tunbridge Wells, Pitman Medical.

Appendix 2.1

Pain arising from the neck, thorax and low back

PAIN ARISING FROM THE NECK AND THORAX

Lying

Whether supine or side-lying, the head/neck should be supported in the neutral position. Down pillows are best (see p. 64).

Supine

Use one pillow to support the neck by shaping the pillow as a 'butterfly' or 'bow tie'. If there is an increased thoracic kyphosis, a folded towel can be placed under the head to prevent an unacceptable degree of craniovertebral extension. Another method is to insert a rolled up small towel inside the pillowcase along the lower border (McKenzie). When any shoulder extension aggravates pain, support the arm with a folded towel underneath.

Side-lying

For those who cannot lie supine, ensure pillows are tucked well in to fill the distance between shoulder cap and neck. With the painful limb uppermost, a pillow between trunk and limb and/or a pillow or folded blanket in front can support and prevent painful 'downdrag'. Very occasionally, lying on the painful side is more comfortable.

Inability to lie low

In order to maintain the neck in neutral, the whole trunk may need to be raised from the waist, using five or six pillows or, more expensively, by an inflatable support placed under the mattress.

Prone

This is particularly stressful and should be avoided. A night collar is usually a deterrent for those who habitually sleep this way.

Sitting

In the acute stage, this may be the only position to give relief. A high-backed accommodating chair with arms is beneficial. The spine, head and arms should be well supported by wearing a soft collar and positioning pillows between limb and chair arm, to relax the shoulder girdle. If the chair back is not high enough to support the head, it can be placed against the wall and another pillow used. A tightly rolled towel behind the lumbar spine (Fig. 2.3) also improves the position of the cervical and thoracic spine. For other modifications see section on seating, pp. 65–67.

Pressure on a hypersensitive thoracic spine can be reduced by long blocks of foam or pillows placed longitudinally up the chair back leaving a gap for the spinous processes. Where an increase in pressure is the relieving factor, a strategically placed hot water bottle is often comforting but patients should be warned to keep the bottle well covered, to avoid burning themselves.

Walking

Use sorbothane heel pads; see below.

PAIN ARISING FROM THE LOW BACK

Supine

Where lying prone or supine either aggravates or does not ease pain, lying supine with the hips and knees flexed is often helpful. The feet and lower legs can be supported by pillows, or on a stool or chair.

Side-lying

This may be more comfortable, perhaps with a pillow between the knees or with the upper leg more flexed and adducted. Alternatively, the lower leg may be drawn up with the upper one extended. A bath sheet rolled lengthwise and wound around the waist helps to support the lumbar spine in neutral, whatever the sleeping position.

Rising

It is usually preferable to encourage the return of the lumber spine's natural lordos before rising. To do this, the patient should be advised to place the hands under the small of the back while lying supine with the knees bent and then very gently move the bent knees a little from side to side before turning on to the side, usually with the more painful limb uppermost, then lower the feet to the floor while pushing up into sitting, keeping the back straight (see Fig. 2.10).

Sitting

Since intradiscal pressure is higher when sitting than in standing and walking and much higher than in lying, this is often the least desirable position. Frequently a lumbar roll (a tightly rolled bath towel; Fig. 2.3), as described by McKenzie, guides the spine into a better position. Patients should be taught how to select the most suitable chair for themselves and how to make adaptations (see section on seating, pp. 65–67).

A temporary toilet seat raise may be helpful.

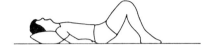

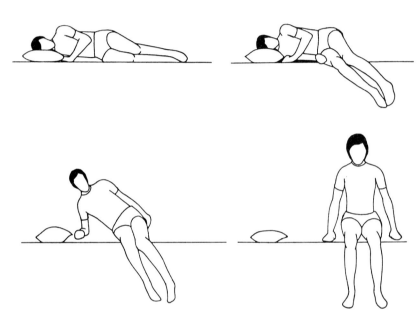

Fig. 2.10 An illustration of the easiest way to adopt the sitting position, placing the minimum amount of strain on the spine. From *You and Your Back*, *Programme 2*, as used in Northwick Park Hospital Department of Rehabilitation

Walking

Keeping steps short and even is usually best. Elbow crutches can reduce the stress on the spine provided they are the correct length and patients do not flex forward on to them.

Sorbothane heel pads

These can help to reduce the jarring of heel strike. They may be bought from sports shops and some large chemists.

Appendix 2.2

Instructions for making a soft collar

Measurements are taken with the head/neck as near to the neutral position as symptoms will allow. These are then transferred to a simple pattern (see Fig. 2.11a) and the collar cut out from 2.5 cm thick foam rubber or similarly dense material. The inner edges should then be bevelled for comfort. The cover is of tubular stockinette. If you are also using this to hold the collar in place, it should be four and a half times the length of the collar, so that it can be wound round twice and tied at the side or

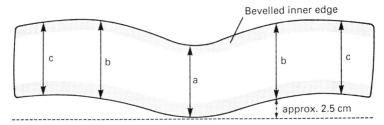

(a) 1. Measure circumference of neck and add 5–7 cm.
     2. Measure:
        a. Below chin to suprasternal notch.
        b. Angle jaw to supraclavicular tissues.
        c. Below occiput to C7.

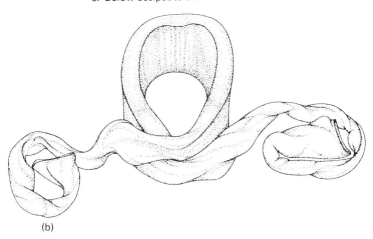

(b)

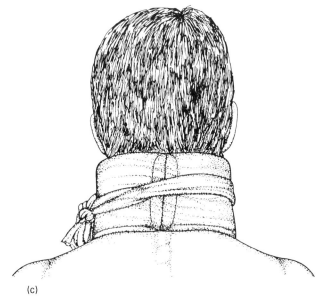

(c)

Fig. 2.11   A pattern for one type of soft collar

front. The stockinette is 'fed' on to the collar from the bottom corner at one end and off it from the top corner at the other, so it can be flattened to cover the free adjacent corner when tying (Fig. 2.11 b and c). If preferred, a velcro band can be used as a tie.

NB: This type of collar does not restrict extension and care should be taken in measuring so that there is no undue pressure on nuchal tissues, as this can cause headaches.

3

Disabling breathlessness

Donald J. Lane

Disability in chest diseases means breathlessness. Breathlessness curtails activity as surely as paralysis or loss of a limb. The patient with severe chest disease may look reassuringly at ease and content sitting in his armchair, but ask him to move a few feet across the room to fetch a newspaper or clear the crockery from the table, and he cannot. The frustration felt by those with severe dyspnoea and their inability to participate in simple everyday activities easily lead to loneliness and despair.

The extent of the health care problem presented by respiratory disability is not known accurately, chiefly because of difficulties in defining degree of disability or in identifying those who are disabled. However some idea of the scale of the problem can be gained by considering the following statistics. Some 10% of all recorded working days lost on account of sickness and some 21% of all general practitioner consultations are attributable to respiratory ill health. Invalidity benefit is paid for respiratory disability to at least 60 000 persons in England and Wales and, whilst only about a third of these are known to receive help with simple tasks of daily living, estimates suggest that up to 330 000 people may have some degree of (often unrecorded) respiratory difficulty; their needs for help could be satisfied but have not yet been identified.

This chapter will examine respiratory disability, that is breathlessness, from the point of view of both mechanisms and management. Much research has been undertaken in an attempt to unravel the mechanisms of dyspnoea, and this will be reviewed. For some, a proper diagnosis can lead to useful therapy for an underlying condition. For others the underlying disease is irreversible. These patients present a challenge that is too often ignored; yet they can be helped and approaches to relieving their distress will be described.

THE CAUSES OF BREATHLESSNESS

A brief survey of the disabling chest diseases

For the purpose of this discussion lung diseases may be grouped under three headings: those that affect the airways, those that infiltrate the parenchyma of the lung, and mass lesions. Mass lesions such as pneumonia, pleural effusion or pneumothorax are acute illnesses nearly always amenable to therapy which dramatically improves the breathlessness with which they present. Pulmonary neoplasia, causing breathlessness from a mass lesion or by widespread infiltration, is regrettably rarely a long-term problem. The healing of infective lesions or the fibrosis that follows radiotherapy for bronchial carcinoma can leave sufficient parenchymal damage to interfere with overall lung function, but widespread fibrosis is more likely to be associated with fibrosing or extrinsic allergic alveolitis, sarcoidosis or certain pneumoconioses. Such patients are greatly distressed by breathlessness, and the functional impairment that gives rise to this is widespread damage to or destruction of lung tissue. But numerically of far greater importance are those disorders that give rise to airways narrowing. Again some, like acute asthma, are reversible. A few asthmatics develop chronic symptoms and so join the multitudes of those with irreversible airways narrowing, most of whom have damaged their lungs smoking cigarettes. Chronic bronchitis is an inadequate term for these sufferers, implying as it does simply cough and sputum production. Such symptoms are annoying and socially distasteful, but they are hardly disabling. It is the chronic irreversible airways narrowing that follows damage to small airways and the insidious destruction of lung units by emphysema that causes their disabling chest disease. Though many terms have been chosen for this condition, perhaps chronic obstructive lung disease is that most used. In addition to these lung disorders consideration may need to be given to breathlessness in patients with thoracic cage disorders. Here muscle weakness is the usual problem and often the breathlessness is only part of a more widespread neuromuscular disorder presenting management problems on a wide front.

It is helpful to think of the problems presented by respiratory diseases (as well as other disabling diseases) on three levels:

1. Functional impairment – the physiologically measurable deficit in lung function which is attributable to the structural changes induced by the disease process.
2. Disability – the effect that functional impairment has on limiting mobility, in this instance by causing breathlessness.
3. Handicap – the impact of disability on the individual's way of life.

Measurement of the impairment in lung function

Functional impairment in chest disease is assessed largely in terms of the mechanical function of the lungs. Simple tests give most information. A full breath from maximum inspiration to maximum expiration delivered into a spirometer will register the vital capacity (VC), an index of the lung size. This expiration is usually delivered with maximum force and the record of the delivery of this volume against time will allow the speed of the forced expiration to be measured. Several indices may be measured from this tracing but that most widely used is the volume expired in one second, the FEV_1. The vital capacity delivered during a forced expiration (FVC) should be similar to that delivered in a more relaxed fashion but in advanced airways disease may be appreciably less. Recorded values for VC and FEV_1 are compared with those for healthy subjects of the same age, sex and height and the ratio of FEV_1:VC (or FEV_1:FVC) is calculated. Normal spirometric function is indicated if results fall within approximately ± 20% of predicted values for VC, FEV_1 and FEV_1:VC: the value of the latter ratio is greater than 70% except in old age.

Two abnormal patterns are defined (see Fig. 3.1 for typical examples):

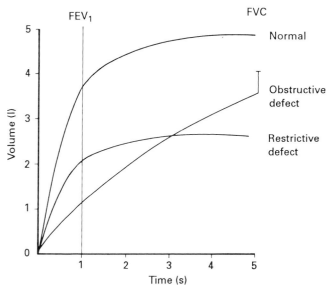

Fig. 3.1 Typical spirometric tracings illustrating normal, restrictive and obstructive patterns. FEV_1 = forced expiratory volume in 1 second; FVC = forced vital capacity

1. A restrictive defect typical of parenchymal lung disease and mass lesions where airways function is normal:
     VC (FVC) reduced
     FEV_1 reduced
     $FEV_1:VC$ within normal limits
2. An obstructive defect, characteristic of airways narrowing:
     VC (FVC) normal or, in advanced disease, reduced
     FEV_1 always reduced
     $FEV_1:VC$ always reduced

A simpler test for airways narrowing which is particularly suited for epidemiological or domiciliary use is the peak expiratory flow. During forced expiration from full inspiration, maximum flow occurs at the very beginning of the breath (Fig. 3.2). Flow meters designed to register peak flow are in common use for the assessment of variable airways narrowing (Fig. 3.3). Parenchymal lung disease causing small lung volumes and any condition causing weakness of the respiratory muscles will also reduce peak expiratory flow, so that the test used alone is not as discriminative as the spirometric recording of VC and FEV_1.

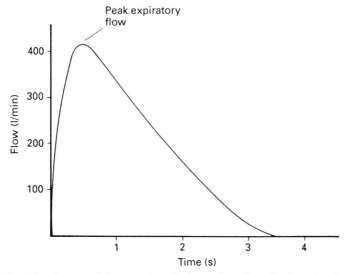

Fig. 3.2   A normal flow tracing during a forced expiration showing peak expiratory flow in early expiration

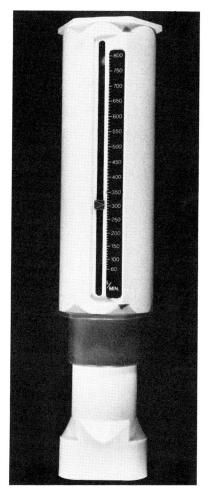

Fig. 3.3   Flow meter for measuring peak expiratory flow

Definition of breathlessness

Breathlessness is ill defined. It is a lay rather than a medical term. None of the medical or physiological terms used in the context of understanding these patients quite covers the sensation felt by patients. Their breathing may be difficult, but dyspnoea is only part of the picture. Their ventilation is increased, certainly, as in the hyperpnoea of exercise, commensurate to their metabolic demands, but also out of proportion to those demands – hyperventilation; and there may be an element of rapid breathing, tachypnoea.

Together all these terms may describe some component of the sensation of breathlessness experienced by patients but none seems totally to qualify as a full description.

In addition, other symptoms crowd in on patients disabled by respiratory disease. They may describe their chests as tight or congested, and cough, whether dry or productive of sputum, may be a distressing additional feature. Disturbed sleep leads to fatigue, loss of memory and irritability. Immobility creates alienation from friends and family and, according to mood and circumstances, anxiety or hopelessness may overwhelm them. Yet behind nearly all this is the central feature of their breathlessness: 'If only I could get my breath, then everything would be all right'.

Mechanisms of breathlessness

Whilst intensive research into the nature of breathlessness has been undertaken in recent years, it is impossible to give an explanation of this symptom that will satisfy all circumstances. Indeed it is highly likely that several mechanisms operate to varying extents in different clinical settings. In order to help the breathless person it is however necessary to have some understanding of the genesis of his or her breathlessness. Any understanding must begin from an appreciation that in health there is a controlled balance between the drive to breathing, the ventilation of the lungs and the metabolic demands of the body.

Exercise breathlessness illustrates this point. When metabolic demands increase during exercise, there is an increased drive to breathing and thus increased ventilation of the lungs sufficient to satisfy the requirements of the exercising muscles for additional oxygen. Except in the later stages of exercise this sensation is not unpleasant to most healthy individuals. When exercise is attempted by those with respiratory illness their dyspnoea is both greater and qualitatively more distressing.

Imbalance between drive and performance

One component of the sensation of respiratory distress that can be deduced from this simple model of respiratory control is an imbalance between the drive to breathe and the performance of the respiratory apparatus. Increased drive can arise in lung disease from hypoxia or from a reflex drive originating in lung receptors stimulated by the pulmonary pathology. Decreased performance will arise because of the mechanical restraints imposed on lung movement by the pathological process, whether it be restrictive disease, stiffening the lung parenchyma, or airways disease increasing resistance of airflow. How this imbalance is perceived is unknown.

Breath-holding

Respiratory distress does not always depend on actual pulmonary movement. A breath-hold is unpleasant even for healthy subjects and is more so for those with most lung disorders. How or whether this component enters into the sensation of breathlessness in disease is not known, but it seems plausible that it may be akin to the sensation experienced by those with thoracic muscle paralysis.

Perception

The sensitivity of cerebral perception is of fundamental importance. The degree of breathlessness recorded at a given level of exercise ventilation varies widely amongst healthy individuals, suggesting wide variations in innate perception. These variations are likely also to influence perceived breathlessness in patients.

Psychogenic factors

Whilst exercise state is the chief precipitant of breathlessness in patients with respiratory disease, it is not the sole one. An increase in cortical activity from anxiety or panic may drive ventilation beyond that necessary for the metabolic requirements of the moment and in doing so cause distress. The low CO_2 which results from excessive hyperventilation leads to multiple symptomatology relating to tissue alkalosis, especially in the nervous system, and alkalosis which further complicates the sensations which trouble the patient. Such patients appear to have breathlessness that is disproportionate to their lung function impairment.

Assessing exercise tolerance

Whatever its exact mechanism, it is the limitation of exercise tolerance by breathlessness that is the disability that afflicts people with breathlessness. Exercise tolerance is thus the yardstick of disability in respiratory disease. Though questionnaires about exercise ability are suitable for epidemiological studies they are not sufficiently reliable for detailed studies of mechanisms or therapy (Table 3.1). Perhaps the simplest objective test is the timed walk. On a flat surface the patient is asked to walk as far as he or she can in a

Table 3.1   Examples of scales of breathlessness

The Medical Research Council breathlessness scale
1. Troubled by shortness of breath when hurrying on level ground or walking up a slight hill.
2. Short of breath when walking with other people of own age on level ground.
3. Have to stop for breath when walking at own pace on level ground.

Classification of acute breathlessness by grade of severity (based on the Jones index)
Grade I   Able to do housework or job with difficulty.
Grade II   Confined to chair/bed but able to get up with moderate difficulty.
Grade IIb   Confined to chair/bed and only able to get up with great difficulty.
Grade III   Totally confined to a chair or bed.
Grade IV   Moribund.

---

specified time, usually 12 minutes. Most studies can be interpreted in terms of total distance walked. The test succeeds because it is easy to perform. There is a learning effect and the measured walking distance only becomes reproducible after several tests. Perhaps one drawback to the test is that it does not push exercise to the limit. In that sense, for the least disabled, it may not stress the respiratory system sufficiently. For these subjects, more formal exercise tolerance tests may be employed and indeed will be relevant over a wide range of disability. These tests, whether using a bicycle ergometer or a treadmill, become more relevant to the question of breathlessness because they do push people to the point of exercise where they must stop because of respiratory distress.

Correlating exercise tolerance with functional impairment

How do indices of disability, as registered by exercise tolerance, correlate with the indices of functional impairment described earlier? Not well. Figure 3.4 illustrates the range and the relationship between total exercise performance by a group of patients with chronic obstructive lung disease and their simultaneously measured airways narrowing, as measured by the FEV_1. Clinical examples highlight the anomalies in this relationship.

Patient A was a thin, gaunt anxious clerk who had retired on account of increasing breathlessness. His overinflated chest was shown to be due to emphysema radiographically. His desperate shortness of breath was reflected in a much reduced exercise tolerance and his airways obstruction quantified by an FEV_1 of 1.0 litres. He is seen from Figure 3.4 to be relatively more short of breath than many other subjects with a similar functional impairment.

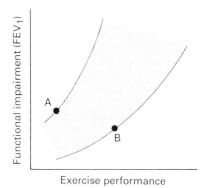

Fig. 3.4   Wide variation in relationship between functional impairment and exercise performance in patients with chronic obstructive lung disease. See text for explanation

Patient B on the other hand was a phlegmatic bricklayer still at work at the age of 57 despite an FEV_1 of 0.65 litres. His exercise tolerance when formally tested was relatively good despite cyanosis, swollen ankles and the stigmata of cor pulmonale. This patient, despite more severe airflow obstruction, was relatively less short of breath.

Two features help to explain the anomalies between these patients and a description of these will pave the way to a discussion of how these patients can be helped.

Adaptation to a complex mechanical problem

The first point is to realize that the FEV_1 is inadequate on its own to express the functional abnormality suffered by these patients with airways obstruction. Patient A had an overinflated chest. Inflation of the lungs requires effort to be expended in stretching the elastic tissues of the lung parenchyma, as in blowing up a balloon. Having to impose on these overinflated lungs the additional effort of breathing in and out is not only very costly in terms of respiratory work, but also distressing as anyone can demonstrate by taking a full breath in and then attempting to move air in and out of the chest. At these high lung volumes it is somewhat easier to achieve a given ventilation by using rapid shallow breaths than by breathing deeply and slowly. This pattern is often adopted by breathless patients with overinflated lungs. Yet, perversely, a pattern of rapid shallow breaths is most costly and one of slow, deep breathing least costly of respiratory effort when narrowing of the airways is the major disease process. 'Choosing' the optimal breathing pattern for least respiratory work under the complex conditions of overinflation with airflow obstruction therefore presents considerable problems. How far there is a genuine choice in a pattern is doubtful: reflex forces undoubtedly contribute significantly to the pattern adopted, though limited voluntary control may be exercised, as will be discussed below.

Individual variation in ventilatory control

The second feature that helps explain the differences between the two patients described concerns ventilatory control. The ventilatory stimulation that follows carbon dioxide (CO_2) accumulation and oxygen lack has been described and extensively studied for over a century. In general, respiratory control mechanisms are more sensitive to small changes in CO_2 pressure (P_{CO_2}) around the physiological level than they are to similar changes in oxygen, but within a group of individuals there will be found a wide range of sensitivities to both gases. Whilst acquired abnormalities of ventilatory control are well documented, it seems likely that there is an inherited ventilatory sensitivity spectrum that may well determine the evolution of disease in individuals. As airways obstruction progresses there comes a point where the reduced airflow leads to inefficient clearance of CO_2. Those born with a high sensitivity to CO_2 will respond vigorously with increased ventilation which, though it prevents CO_2 retention, accentuates the dyspnoea. Patient A above is an example of this and it is easy to see why he has the nickname, the 'pink puffer'. Others with poor CO_2 sensitivity will not respond with increased ventilation, will tend to accumulate CO_2, but relatively speaking, will be less short of breath for a given degree of functional impairment (Patient B above). These patients look cyanosed, and develop ankle oedema due to cor pulmonale, thus earning their nickname, the 'blue bloater'.

Yet these physiologically based considerations do not satisfactorily explain all the differences in disability encountered amongst patients with chronic obstructive lung disease. The most important additional factor lies in the psyche. In attempts to analyse those features which determine disability as measured by the 12-minute walking test, assessments of certain attitudes and beliefs proved more important than tests of functional impairment. These assessments, based on recognized psychological techniques, showed that the patients' perception of the amount of exertion required was of the greatest importance, and also that distance walked was further if they had confidence in the treatment offered but shorter if they thought their bronchitis was 'bad'.

Taken together then, mechanical adaptation to airways narrowing, innate ventilatory drives, perception and belief all combine and interact in producing respiratory disability. Though complex, it has been necessary to outline the issues involved in the genesis of respiratory disability in order to provide some of the background for a discussion of the potential for helping people with disabling breathlessness.

THERAPEUTIC APPROACHES

The relief of disabling breathlessness in those with respiratory disorders may be considered under the following headings:

1. Treatment of the underlying condition.
2. Modification of the mechanical problems.
3. Depression of abnormal ventilatory drive.
4. Modification of central perception.
5. General approach to exercise.

Treatment of the underlying condition

It is almost trite to begin any discussion of therapeutic management in disabled people by stating that the underlying condition must be treated wherever possible. This approach needs emphasizing in relation to chronic lung disease because reversible components, especially in airways disease, masquerade as or accompany an apparently irreversible condition. It is easy to dismiss the disabling breathlessness of the middle-aged smoker as all due to his chronic obstructive bronchitis, but it is important to pick out the reversible component in the history by asking about childhood asthma or other atopic disease, or a family history of the same; to attempt to detect atopy with skinprick testing and sputum or blood eosinophilia, and to look for reversibility to bronchodilators, or with serial peak flow measurements to reveal the tell-tale morning dip of the asthmatic (Fig. 3.5). If any of these assessments give clues that there may be reversibility of the airways obstruction then it is important to institute a steroid trial, details of which are given in Table 3.2.

Even when there is no steroid reversibility some response may still be obtained from bronchodilator therapy alone. Beta$_2$ stimulants are the accepted first approach and sometimes the larger doses, which are possible by using nebulizers, may succeed where conventional pressurized aerosols have been ineffective. For the bronchitic type of patient parasympathomimetic drugs are often as good as or even better than beta$_2$ stimulants.

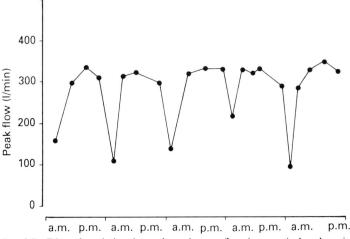

Fig. 3.5 Diurnal variation in peak expiratory flow in a typical asthmatic patient

Atropine itself is seldom used now but ipratropium, either alone in a pressurized aerosol (Atrovent), or in combination with the beta$_2$ stimulant fenoterol (Duovent) has found a useful place in the management of these patients. Xanthines (aminophylline, theophylline) unfortunately quite often give gastrointestinal upset but if well tolerated and used in adequate dose to obtain therapeutic levels in the blood will add not only an element of bronchodilatation but also possibly a biochemical advantage in increasing respiratory muscle efficiency. Very often only a part of the airways obstruction will be reversible but nonetheless even a small improvement in airways function may lead to a very worthwhile improvement in exercise tolerance.

In interstitial lung disease there is usually less room for manoeuvre. Certain conditions do respond to steroids or even cytotoxics but whether or

Table 3.2   Steroid trial protocol

Assess with twice-daily peak flow

Record baseline data for 1–2 weeks

Treat with prednisolone 15 mg b.d.

After 1 week reassess:
  positive if > 20% increase in peak flow
  if negative, continue for second week

If still negative, patient's airways obstruction is not steroid-responsive not these are employed will depend on a detailed knowledge of the type of disorder, possibly with pulmonary histology. Regrettably parenchymal disease is often irreversibly fibrotic.

Modification of the mechanical problems

Breathing exercises which aim to relieve breathlessness have a time-honoured, if controversial, place in the management of a patient with respiratory disease. Once again, and largely because of the numerical problem, patients with chronic obstructive lung disease have received the most attention. It is important to realize from the outset that breathing exercises cannot influence the underlying disease. There is no voluntary control over bronchial smooth muscle. So what can breathing exercises offer? A way of breathing that may help the patient with airways obstruction to cope with the difficulties that are the consequence of airways narrowing and with the sense of tension and panic that so often overwhelms them.

There are two principles which underlie breathing exercises in airways obstruction. These are relaxation and control: relaxation of tension, not only in the muscles that move the chest but muscles throughout the body: control over panic, as well as control over the breathing muscles themselves. Some comments on general relaxation will be made below: this section will concentrate on the breathing exercises themselves. Analyses of breathing patterns suggest that patients with airflow obstruction often breathe too quickly. It has been explained that this is costly in the presence of airways obstruction, though it may help cope to some extent with severe over-inflation. In general, patients with airflow obstruction must be taught to breathe more slowly. Objective measurements have shown that slowing the rate of breathing in these patients will produce a more efficient gas exchange. Control of the rate of breathing must be taught when the patient's chest is in a stable state so that the technique may be employed in moments of panic and anxiety. A few patients learn to slow down expiration for themselves by using the trick known as pursed-lip breathing: by half closing the lips the flow of air out of the lungs is slowed down.

Much has been said in the past about emptying the lungs 'properly'. There was some logic in this since breathing with hyperinflated lungs is certainly very uncomfortable, but for many patients with airflow obstruction this means that the already narrowed airways are made even narrower by a forced expiration, which only makes things worse. Patients should be encouraged to allow the lungs to relax to the natural endpoint of the breath, and then gently and unhurriedly take the next breath in.

A belief has long existed that it is possible independently to move one part of the chest rather than another. Though it is unlikely that anyone can learn to move one side of the chest independently of the other, there is evidence that concentrating on upper chest movement as opposed to lower chest movement is possible. The concentration on lower chest movement is usually discussed under the heading of diaphragmatic or abdominal–diaphragmatic breathing. Movement down of the diaphragm is encouraged by allowing the anterior abdominal wall to relax forwards. Such a breathing technique can be taught and there is evidence that it relieves breathlessness, especially when combined with slowing the rate of breathing.

In advanced airways obstruction because the diaphragm starts from a very flat position there is sometimes a paradoxical movement of the abdominal wall inwards with inspiration. This is probably no more than a mechanical consequence of the severe airflow obstruction but there is some suggestion that it may be an acquired 'bad breathing habit'. Such patients often find a crouching position relieves acute distress, presumably by forcing the diaphragm into a more domed position.

Recent research has thrown considerable light on diaphragmatic function but has also raised an interesting paradox. The central issue lies in whether the diaphragm needs resting because it becomes fatigued or whether it should be deliberately exercised in order to increase its strength. Perhaps it is more a question of when each of these applies rather than one being correct to the exclusion of the other. In acute respiratory failure resting the diaphragm may indeed help it to recover, whereas in a more chronic stable state, techniques (such as blowing or sucking against resistances) to strengthen the diaphragm may well be more apppropriate. Certain drugs, such as the theophyllines, increase diaphragmatic contractility and perhaps some of their beneficial effect is due to their effect on the diaphragm rather than their action as bronchodilators.

The rules about the control of the rate of breathing and the use of the diaphragm apply especially to breathing during walking and other physical exertion. Various timing instructions are recommended. The exact details are probably unimportant, the essential point being to teach rhythmic breathing in time with the steps taken. Two commonly recommended patterns are to breathe out for two steps and in for one step or to breathe out for three steps and in for two steps.

Depression of abnormal ventilatory drive

Though theoretically this could be a useful approach, in practice ventilatory depression has serious limitations. Ventilatory control is critical in many of these patients and the abolition of a drive may only serve to depress ventilation to such a degree that CO_2 retention follows. The use of morphia or heroin, though valuable in acute pulmonary oedema, is for the most part contraindicated in patients with chronic obstructive lung disease. Trials with the relatively weak opiate dihydrocodeine have been reported, but with disappointing results. Some patients do report somewhat less dyspnoea, but an overall rather weak effect together with constipation mean that this approach cannot be recommended.

Though not strictly speaking a therapy designed to diminish ventilatory drive, the use of hypothyroid drugs may be considered here. There is depression of the response to the chemical drives – hypercapnia and hypoxia – in hypothyroidism, but the use of drugs such as carbimazole was originally proposed on the grounds that it would reduce metabolic requirements for oxygen and so reduce demand on the lungs. This approach has not been successful.

On the other hand the use of oxygen to counteract undue ventilatory stimulation from hypoxia cannot be so lightly dismissed. In the person with distressing breathlessness and severe hypoxia due to diffuse pulmonary fibrosis, oxygen is almost mandatory. It is without danger in these patients but regrettably not always as beneficial as might be hoped, since part of the ventilatory drive comes from pulmonary reflexes rather than from hypoxia. On the other hand pure oxygen can be as dangerous as opiates in the patient with chronic obstructive lung disease and poor CO_2 sensitivity who is reliant on hypoxia to maintain reasonable ventilation. The greatest danger is in the acute setting when the injudicious use of oxygen can set in train a potentially fatal sequence of hypoventilation and worsening gas exchange. For these patients 24% or 28% oxygen is essential, though even these small additions can sometimes be dangerous. Retention of CO_2 occurs less readily in the stable patient but can still occur. Oxygen is rarely needed in this context to relieve dyspnoea: indeed these patients with chronic actual or incipient CO_2 retention are often not greatly troubled by dyspnoea (as in patient B above, the 'blue bloater'). Continuous (at least 15 h/day) low-flow oxygen therapy can be, and is, used to ward off the hypoxic complications of cor pulmonale and secondary polycythaemia, and in this sense may be regarded as a measure against serious and disabling consequences of chronic obstructive lung disease. The technical and social problems of delivering this amount of oxygen in the home using cylinders can now be overcome. The DHSS have agreed that oxygen concentrators (which extract oxygen from ambient air and are run on electricity) are a cost-effective delivery system, and are now prescribable.

The use of oxygen to relieve breathlessness in patients with chronic obstructive lung disease who are not significantly hypoxic is more controversial. The facts are that patients report relief of distressing dyspnoea, especially in the recovery phase after exertion, and they also perform better if they breathe oxygen during exercise. The cylinder standing beside the patient's chair at home may seem to be offering little more than a placebo effect but in some ill understood way it does help these very breathless, often emphysematous, patients to cope with life at home.

Modification of central perception

The very breathless patient is so clearly distressed by his or her condition, and so often anxious about his or her inability to move about, that it is hardly surprising that tranquillizers in various guises have been tried. The opiates, already mentioned, are one group. In the very breathless, pink and puffing patient with a normal or reduced CO_2 tension a cautious trial can be justified. Careful watch must be kept on blood gases and pre-emptive laxatives should be used to avoid the distress of constipation. Anxiolytic drugs, which have minimal effect on ventilatory control, have not proved of much benefit. After one encouraging report of a useful reduction in breathlessness from diazepam in emphysematous, pink and puffing patients, subsequent trials have been disappointing. Promethazine has some effect in reducing the perception of breathlessness in normal subjects but again has not gained a place in the treatment of patients. There is one report of short term benefit from Traditional Chinese Acupuncture in breathless patients with chronic airways obstruction. Exercise tolerance improved but not lung function, so presumably this was an effect in perception.

General approach to exercise

Simple exercise training to maintain tone and mobility in arms and legs has a twofold role in the rehabilitation of those with severe respiratory disorders. First, by improving general muscle power and fitness exercise tolerance is increased to the limits allowed by lung capacity; secondly, by the repeated performance of simple exercise tasks the fear of breathlessness is overcome. Altering attitudes towards exertion by encouragement and by demonstrating to the patient what he or she can do has a vital role in exercise rehabilitation. Integral to both of these are tactical points about exercise training specific to patients with respiratory problems – taking tasks slowly, interspersing effort with frequent stops so that much greater distances can be achieved, taking stairs one at a time, relaxing fully during stops and using breathing techniques and ambulatory oxygen, as described earlier. Above all, in exercise training for respiratory disability as in so many other areas of rehabilitation it is hard work, repetition and motivation that achieve results – on the part of patients and staff alike.

HANDICAP AS A RESULT OF RESPIRATORY DISABILITY

The features which influence the translation of disability into handicap are similar whatever the disability. Severe breathlessness can deprive a farm-worker of his livelihood as surely as extensive rheumatoid arthritis, yet the office-worker need not suffer the handicap of losing his or her job from either of these disabling diseases. Provision of suitable transport, building adaptation and gaining the co-operation of employers are essential considerations in the task of limiting the handicap resulting from respiratory disability. Those already in sedentary occupations find it easier to adapt to increasing limitation of their exercise tolerance by breathlessness and so manage to stay at work longer. Simple adjustments to office routine can minimize the need for move-ment from place to place. Most sufferers from severe breathlessness will re-main able to drive a car long after they cease to be able to walk very far and a privileged parking place close to the works entrance is a small consideration for continued employment. The disabled parking disc will help at other times, though it is always difficult to define the degree of breathlessness that should qualify one for this concession: perhaps inability to walk 100 yards would be reasonable but it would also be arbitrary and arguable.

For those in manual occupations the situation is more difficult. Within a large organization the worker with respiratory disability can be moved to pro-gressively less arduous jobs, hopefully still using his or her experience but de-creasing the need to move about or lift heavy objects. Many finish up in advisory posts. Others are supported by fellow workers long after they have become physically incapable of carrying out the tasks normally expected of them. Those whose work performs an important role in a small organization fare worse than those carrying out a small task in a large organization.

A rehabilitation course may be able to train such patients for more sedent-ary occupations, though in today's economic climate eventual hopes of em-ployment are bleak. Employment rehabilitation centres are run by the Training Commission with some help from the Employment Medical Advis-ory Service, a medical branch of the Department of Employment. Some 5% of those attending these courses have respiratory disability. This is not a high figure and until recently the problems of patients with respiratory dis-ability have not featured prominently in the consideration or successes of this service. Drop-out rate has been higher for respiratory cases than for others. The reasons for disappointment with the re-employment services are complex. Patients are often referred late in their illness or have educational qualifications that do not fit them well for a sedentary occupation. By comparison with patients having limb or joint disorders, patients with respiratory disease do not look upon themselves as 'disabled'; they are also often disturbed by the smoking habits of others in the rehabilitation centre.

Any approach to helping the respiratory cripple retain or regain employment must take cognizance of the very strong psychological component to breathlessness. Several studies have shown that attitude and motivation are of fundamental importance. They determine the willingness both to tolerate situations which cause breathlessness and to persevere with exercises designed to help them cope with breathlessness. Prospectively, within a group of severely disabled bronchitics, it was psychological parameters which determined time off work during the year of observation rather than physiological measurements related to functional impairment or disability. Those who were depressed, those who viewed life negatively and who looked upon their work as hard or difficult lost more time from work than those who had more positive attitudes.

PROVIDING EFFECTIVE HELP

The problems of the respiratory cripple were highlighted in the report *Disabling Chest Disease: Prevention and Care*.[1] The Committee of the Royal College of Physicians saw unfulfilled needs at several stages in the life history of those patients who became respiratory cripples. In prevention the primary problem was seen as the identification of those patients likely to become disabled at a stage when they are relatively healthy. Minor deviations from normal lung function found in middle-aged smokers predict an increased risk of eventual disability. Such changes could be detected by regular health checks, through population surveys, in general practitioner surgeries or at the workplace. The action necessary, once a suspicion of future trouble has been detected, is to secure a change in lifestyle that would remove risk factors. For the most part this means an aggressive campaign to stop the patient smoking – and in some instances may entail altering working conditions where pollution is a problem.

Symptomatic illness in these patients begins insidiously and there is a general impression amongst the public that bronchitis is not serious. Regrettably, once breathlessness has become part of the clinical picture much irreversible damage to the lungs has already been sustained. Even at this stage there seems to be an ignorance concerning what measures can be used to help, and a low expectation for successful outcome. These impressions are not confined to the patient but unfortunately extend to nurses, general practitioners and hospital doctors, whose task it should be to provide care and prevent decline in health. The reasons for these observations are manifold. Partly it is in the nature of the progressive, largely irreversible, obstructive lung disease; partly it is knowledge that the condition is to a significant extent self-induced; partly it is that cough and sputum are socially distasteful and breathlessness socially isolating. Furthermore, no pressure group exists to fight for the disabled bronchitic in the way the Diabetic Association or the Multiple Sclerosis Society supports the needs of victims of these disorders.

Day care

For the most severely disabled individual, employment is no longer an option and life becomes a bitter struggle to survive and overcome the isolation of immobility. Considerate friends and caring relatives can do much to alleviate the loneliness and helplessness of the respiratory cripple especially in closely knit, usually rural communities, but when friends have gone and the family is small and scattered care must be provided on a communal basis. For the past few years the Chest Unit in Oxford has run a day unit for these patients. The unit is staffed by occupational therapists, with volunteer help from the League of Friends. Being situated close to the rest of the clinical chest department, the unit has the support of nursing, medical and physiotherapy staff. Patients attend once a week for a full day – diversional occupational therapy from printing to toy-making, cooking to gardening provides tasks easy to perform even for the most breathless. Visitors entertain or demonstrate in the winter months and outings in a minibus provide highlights in better weather. The obvious enjoyment of the participants and the gratitude of the spouse relieved of responsibility even for just a day are sufficient to justify the time and effort put into the unit even without formal assessments of cost-effectiveness.

The person very severely handicapped from chest disease often suffers from neglect and isolation that are not deserved. The care of these patients represents a real challenge and one that many more units could take up. Whilst the ultimate hope is that prevention, especially by reducing smoking, will make this a numerically unimportant problem, some patients with respiratory disability will always be with us, requiring the provision of services to help them live with their particular disability.

REFERENCE

1. Royal College of Physicians of London (1981), Disabling chest disease; prevention and care *J. R. Coll. Med.*; **15**: 69–87.

4

Coronary rehabilitation

Elizabeth Yates

INTRODUCTION

This book has explored some conditions in which adjustments have to be made by individuals and their families to disabilities, the majority of which are easily recognized visually. Coronary artery disease does not have visually overt stigmata or impairments such as joint deformities. This lack of obvious signs of illness leads to confusion in lay people. Their intentions of responding positively to an individual with coronary artery disease often lead to over-protection. This absence of overt disability also has an effect upon the victim, in whom the sudden onset of a life-threatening illness such as a myocardial infarction can have devastating psychological effects leading to acute anxiety and complete loss of confidence.

This anxiety and loss of confidence is well founded since coronary heart disease is the single largest cause of death in Britain today; furthermore it has been demonstrated that the prevalence of coronary heart disease in one form or another in individuals age 40–44 years is 17.6%, rising to 31.2% in the 55–59 year age group. It is estimated that one man in ten in the age range 55–59 will manifest the disease in a severe form. Acute myocardial infarction is perhaps the best known manifestation of this condition and is certainly the one which calls for rehabilitation. It is estimated that there are 35 000 acute infarctions among males aged 40–59 years in England and Wales every year, and that two out of every five of these episodes occur in the age range 55–59 years. While these figures are of great concern they disguise the fact that a large number of patients who have suffered an acute myocardial infarction are able to lead normal lives and frequently have no further manifestations of the underlying condition for a number of years. Rehabilitation is most important for these people since their prognosis is good and the older attitudes of prolonged invalidism have been shown to be unnecessary.

All general practitioners have patients in their care following myocardial infarction. This chapter outlines the need for careful explanation and education about this condition and some methods by which patients can be helped to understand what has happened to them, together with a programme aimed at the restoration of confidence. Reports from the World Health Organization[1,2] have stressed the importance of rehabilitation following myocardial infarction enabling people to achieve their optimum function in all occupational and/or environmental areas of their life.

The essential ingredient of any successful programme is a coherent team supervising and implementing its operation. This team must share information, common goals and policy of care. Conflict should be reduced to a minimum and when it exists should not be extended to the patient or family. The team should include all health personnel providing services to patients both in hospital and at home. The family and employers, or their representatives, must be involved. The inclusion of the family and employer as team members improves the opportunity for factual information and advice to be exchanged and should reduce the level of protection developed by family, friends and colleagues towards the patient.

It is appreciated that not everybody who has a myocardial infarction will be treated in hospital. The principles of rehabilitation following a cardiac infarction remain the same whether the initial phase of management is at home or in hospital. Consequently no further reference will be made to the management of patients at home. Where a good hospital-based programme exists, however, many general practitioners are happy to make use it.

HOSPITAL MANAGEMENT OF THE ACUTE STAGE

The rehabilitation process should commence on admission to hospital. Although the patient may be in no condition to appreciate diagnostic or treatment details, relatives and friends accompanying the patient require information and, when appropriate, reassurance. Although not all patients read leaflets, information relating to diagnosis, medication and investigations should be provided continually during hospitalization and after care. Many units now publish their own information leaflets for patients and relatives. These leaflets reflect the unit's policy of care and describe the disease, its aetiology and epidemiology. Separate leaflets describe specific investigations such as angiography and dietary advice.

The Chest, Heart and Stroke Association (see Chapter 14) publish a number of leaflets which may be of use in the absence of local publications. Some food manufacturers, e.g. Flora, also produce advice leaflets. Leaflets published by other groups should be checked before introduction to a unit to ensure that the information they provide does not conflict with the policy of the unit.

Admission to a coronary care unit creates dependence. Human and electronic monitors assume responsibility for the patient's well-being. Few significant decisions are made by the patient even at the level of personal maintenance, e.g. clothing or bathing. Modern policies of rapid mobilization and resumption of toilet activities without resource to the bedpan or the bedside commode are of enormous importance in re-establishing patient confidence and rapidly identify those patients in whom the prognosis may be expected to be impaired and further manifestations of the disease are likely to ensue. Transfer to the ward environment begins the preparation for discharge. Staffing levels are reduced and the patient is gradually given back responsibility for self-maintenance, such as personal decision-making and activities relating to personal hygiene, feeding, dressing and mobility. Nursing supervision is withdrawn as the patient's medical state stabilizes and his or her physical ability increases. Mobilization outside the ward is usually supervised by physiotherapists and will include supervised practice of climbing stairs.

In most hospitals patients now undergo a formal exercise test on a supervised treadmill with electrocardiographic monitoring which is designed to identify those in whom further complications may be expected or those whose prognosis is good. This is a very important part of rehabilitation since the exercise is usually maximal and takes place under strictly controlled and medically supervised conditions which instil a great deal of confidence.

A detailed history of the patient's pre-coronary lifestyle, social and domestic work is of value at this stage, associated with a description of his or her living accommodation and local environment. This information will be used during the rehabilitation programme for structuring advice in conjunction with his or her level of function and the extent of the disease.

The occupational therapist will use this information when advising on post-discharge activities. The ergonomics and sequencing of routine domestic activities will be discussed with the patient and if possible with the spouse or other family members. Therapists and nurses should verbally reinforce the observation by relatives of the patient's performance of self-maintenance activities during visits, demonstrating that it is no longer necessary for things to be done for the patient. Relatives' acceptance of the patient's functioning independently on the ward is essential if over-protective behaviour at home is to be prevented or reduced.

Additional information is required by the family prior to discharge from hospital. This is usually in response to questions which commence 'What do I do if. . . ?' Verbal reinforcement of leaflets such as *Coronary After Care* by the Chest, Heart and Stroke Association (Chapter 14) will reduce anxiety. Local procedures for medical and emergency services should be clarified. The patient's response to various signs and symptoms is discussed and clarified, e.g. when to rest and have medication, call the doctor or ambulance etc.

OUTPATIENT REHABILITATION PROGRAMME

The outpatient rehabilitation programme should fulfill three criteria:

1. Enable the patient to acknowledge the diagnosis of coronary artery disease, know the risk factors and have the ability to modify individual risks.
2. Enable the patient to increase physical activity in monitored and functional environments.
3. Facilitate the return to a normal diurnal pattern of life.

Such a programme may be provided on either a group or an individual basis. The interaction and self-help nature of group programmes appears to promote the return of self-confidence and independence. When a programme is performed in a clinical environment (which is essential if an exercise component is included), adequate resuscitation facilities must be available. Few programmes contain the full range of possible components – relaxation, discussion, exercise and functional or practical activities – but tend to polarize at either exercise or discussion and relaxation. Either should allow the redevelopment of a normal daily pattern of activities at different paces. The ideal programme should extend over the greater part of a working day, avoiding rush-hour travel, and all components must include the ability of patients to perform at their own pace. An illustrative programme is outlined in Tables 4.1 and 4.2.

The outpatient programme, whatever its component parts, should be dis-

Table 4.1 Example of timetable of a coronary rehabilitation programme

10.00–11.00	Graded activities
11.00–11.30	Graded exercises
11.30–12.30	Support group
	(spouses group meets monthly)
12.30–13.30	Lunch
13.30–14.00	Relaxation
14.00–14.30	Graded group games
14.30–15.15	Graded activities

Table 4.2   Example of an individual programme resulting in gradually increasing physical exertion

Activity	Task	Grading
Printing	Typesetting Type dissing	*Seated* Initially type tray lifted by staff, later lifted by patient
	Use of guillotine and use of press	Standing and sitting
	All aspects of printing	Moving at will doing all relevant lifting and carrying
Woodwork	Sanding Painting Planing	General mobility Activities timed
	General bench work High-speed tools Foot-powered lathe	Rest at will

cussed with the patient and family prior to discharge from hospital. Information relating to site and extent of infarction, pulse rate and blood pressure on discharge, medication and follow-up arrangements should be available to the therapist organizing and supervising the rehabilitation programme.

Transport to enable the individual to attend the rehabilitation programme is important and should be confirmed prior to hospital discharge. Until permission to restart driving is given by the doctor responsible for the patient's care, transport must be provided by either the family or the unit organizing the programme. On group-organized programmes, spouses may take turns to provide transport for small groups of (two to three) people.

It is a requirement of British law that disabilities affecting an individual's fitness to drive should be reported to the Driver and Vehicle Licensing Centre in Swansea (Chapter 14) if the effect of the disability lasts, or is expected to last for more than 8 weeks. There is a blanket recommendation that no patient should resume driving for 6 weeks after an acute myocardial infarction but this should not be interpreted too literally. For many patients the signal that things have returned to normal is permission to drive their car again and there is no reason why a patient who has suffered an uncomplicated myocardial infarct, does not have angina and had a negative exercise test on discharge should not be quite safe to resume control of his or her vehicle within 2 weeks of discharge. Motor insurance companies, however, usually request information on any complications which may affect a driver's ability to drive, however temporary the condition. Failure to inform such an insurer may invalidate a policy, therefore patients should be advised to notify their motor insurance company. If notification follows permission by the doctor to restart driving they should give the doctor's name, date and place of the consultation.

Meal times during the programme may be used therapeutically. Dietary advice is usually available to all patients during hospitalization. Patients may be given the lunch options available at work. Use of the canteen facilities available in a hospital, or packed lunches from home, enables them to return to a 'normal' behaviour pattern. In a community setting small snack bars, pubs or restaurants may be adjacent to the rehabilitation unit. The choice of food despite dietary advice will ultimately rest with the patient.

PSYCHOLOGICAL MANAGEMENT

The psychological impact of myocardial infarction is often the most disabling factor of the disease. Negative and positive responses have been described. Either the patient denies the diagnosis of myocardial infarction, medication and aftercare advice, or totally accepts it together with the perceived handicap and dependence expected with this diagnosis. Some of the handicap may be attributed to an anxiety response to a 'loss of health', as one patient described his feelings, or bereavement. Indeed, the rejection, anger, bargaining and acceptance sequence associated with bereavement may be observed in patients as they come to terms with their disease.

Anxiety management regimens, support or counselling groups associated with relaxation sessions are appropriate techniques which enable the patient to resolve anxieties and the therapist to modify inappropriate behaviour and provide advice. The therapist who organizes this section of the rehabilitation programme should have both training and experience in group dynamics and management, as well as a knowledge of coronary artery disease. Regular supervision sessions should also be available to the therapist.

Patients share a number of anxieties relating to lifestyle, diet, work and sex. A fundamental aspect of rehabilitation is the pre-emption of these anxieties and this may be clearly manifested to the patient by his or her ability to perform physical activities and by discussion groups which must be shared with the patient's spouse. Many wives are frightened to leave their husbands alone at any time and many men have an equal fear. Counselling and reassurance on this point are vital if normal life is to be resumed.

The lifestyle question may be introduced by patients as a complaint, or a description of over-protective attitudes at home. Some spouses stay home to look after the patient, relieving them of all domestic and personal tasks. This results in making the patient dependent and is not therapeutic. Comparisons with social histories taken prior to discharge will confirm unnecessary changes to pre-coronary routines.

Some male patients attempt to manipulate the domestic situation. They may use their real or imagined loss of physical tolerance to stop such domestic tasks as washing up, laundry and meal preparation. This is most likely if the man feels that it is inappropriate for men to be doing domestic work. It may be seen where both the husband and wife work when the chores were previously shared between them.

MANAGEMENT OF RISK FACTORS

Smoking

Smoking is a recognized risk factor associated with coronary artery disease. All patients who smoke are advised to stop following identification of the disease. For some the trauma of a myocardial infarction provides the necessary incentive. The return to the smoking environment following discharge will increase the withdrawal difficulties for most patients. The group gives support for its members and reinforces the advice given to help overcome withdrawal symptoms in the initial period of non-smoking. The introduction of alternative activities such as worry beads is of value to some individuals in this situation.

Diet

Eating is sometimes used as an alternative activity to smoking. Patients claim that food tastes better after a while, their appetite improves and this may be accompanied by a weight increase. Dietary advice is required on suitable food for 'nibbles'. Nuts, sweets and grapes are contra-indicated, whilst raw carrots and apples are suggested.

Low cholesterol and reducing diets may be recommended for specific patients. These may be expensive to implement for patients on low incomes and this factor should be taken into account when preparing diet sheets.

The familial aspect of coronary artery disease makes it important to advise families to introduce a health-conscious attitude to food selection and preparation. The Health Education Authority (Chapter 14) publishes a number of leaflets on this topic and most health authorities are now developing healthy eating policies available to local health personnel.

The preparation of food also makes a difference. Steaming, grilling, or roasting on a rack over a pan are all methods of reducing fat content while cooking, as compared with frying which increases the fat content. Menu planning and meal preparation are activities which may be carried over to the functional activity component of the programme by the occupational therapist and dietitian. This session should demonstrate alternative methods of preparing imaginative and healthy meals.

Alcohol, like smoking, creates problems for those individuals who drank excessively prior to infarction. A glass of wine with a meal or a measure of spirit in the evening will do no harm. A large consumption of alcohol, beer, wine or spirit is not advised and may also result in a weight increase.

RESETTLEMENT

Employment

A number of reports from England and abroad record a low return to work by patients following infarction. Job loss given the present economic situation is a genuine fear. There also appears to be a trend in employers to encourage patients to take early retirement and a reluctance to employ people with a history of coronary artery disease. This may be counteracted in two ways. Firstly, a return to work should be as early as possible (6–10 weeks depending on the severity of infarction and its associated complications). Secondly, the employer should be included as a member of the extended remedial team whenever possible.

The Disablement Resettlement Officer (DRO; see also pp. 61, 95–6, 132–3) will provide the links with employers on the patient's behalf. Some driving and all flying licences become invalid if the holder of such a licence has had a myocardial infarction. Drivers of trains, buses, lorries and coaches, as well as pilots are consequently unable to return to their jobs. When such patients are identified early contact should be made with their employers or their occupational health department. The identification of alternative jobs using the past skills and experience of the individual with the same employer is the first objective. Should this fail, the information in the job history will be of use for the DRO when seeking alternative jobs and/or retraining. This is an integral part of the rehabilitation programme.

Patients' other anxieties related to work are about time and task planning and doubts over their ability to say 'No' to colleagues and bosses at work should they feel tired. Ergonomic advice coupled with assertion techniques should help to reduce their fears and increase confidence.

Marital, sexual and family relationships

Relationships within the family also cause anxiety. Some patients have described a lowered noise tolerance which demonstrates itself in irritation to small dogs yapping and the noise of young children. Over-protection of previously active persons seems to increase this anxiety and makes counselling of relatives important.

Fear of excess activity and its potential fatal result causes anxiety relating to the restarting of sexual relationships. Few patients will initiate discussion of this personal topic and it is essential that the therapist should give 'permission' to the group for its introduction.

The energy expenditure during sexual activity has been related to climbing a flight of stairs, or walking briskly (at approximately 4 miles per hour). These benchmarks give patients a practical guide to their physical activity and may reduce their initial fears. There are, however, some exceptions; familiar partners and environments are less stressful than sexual activity with new partners and new situations. Ergonomic advice relating to positions used during sexual activity should also be provided.

Other factors may also delay or prohibit the return to normal sexual activity. Surveys have demonstrated an almost uniform decrease in sexual activity amongst middle-aged men after a first myocardial infarction. There may be good reasons for this, but the decrease is so universal that it is almost as though many men use the event as an excuse to cease sexual activity altogether. Loss of libido may be drug-induced (by beta-blockers) and some patients experience impotence. These symptoms should be identified and discussed with the physician. It may be necessary if impotence persists to refer the patient for sexual counselling at a psychosexual clinic. Drug-induced reduction in libido may require changes to medication, although spontaneous correction does occur.

Occasionally the return to normal sexual relationships may be hindered by a reluctance on the part of the spouse – the 'healthy' partner. Wives are known to have used the husband's coronary episode to end painful sexual activity caused by menopausal gynaecological changes. Identification of the real reason, followed by appropriate treatment for the wife removes this barrier.

It is difficult to exclude the family and more specifically the spouse or partner from discussions. Many of the patients' anxieties and fears relate to and involve the family. Support groups for spouses both alone and together with their partner provide opportunities to continue the educational component of the programme.

Physical management

Many of the questions raised by patients and relatives relate to physical activities – can they be done, and if so how much? There is a need to know how to recognize danger signals. The activity components of the programme enable therapists to demonstrate answers to these questions and teach patients to monitor themselves – the final acceptance of responsibility for themselves. Every effort should be made to encourage patients to resume normal activities as soon as possible and it should be pointed out that their performance on the rehabilitation course is a good indicator of what they can or cannot do. Rigid rules should be avoided as much as possible and patients must be encouraged to find out for themselves what they can or cannot do. There is a wide misconception that vigorous physical activity precipitates myocardial infarction but there is now ample evidence to show that this is not the case. Most myocardial infarctions occur during the morning and most frequently at breakfast time and it would appear that the events which precipitated the infarction are very seldom related to intense physical activity. There is no evidence at all to suggest that physical activity causes long-term deterioration in the state of the damaged heart. On the contrary, it is more likely that continued activity will maintain myocardial tone and vigour and will certainly enhance the quality of life in these patients.

Exercises and games

The first section of this component is exercise and games supervised by the physiotherapist (Fig. 4.1a). Patients may be taught to record their pulse rate and this is checked before and after each exercise. New exercises begin when the resting pulse is achieved. Exercised muscle requires less oxygen than flabby muscle. All patients are therefore encouraged to take part in this component and to introduce regular exercise into their post-rehabilitation weekly routine.

Exercises are graded by time, frequency of performance or resistance. Included in this section are measured walks, step-ups and cycling (fixed speed and resistance). Some may progress to more active equipment such as the rowing machine. This section of the physiotherapy programme is carried out on an individual basis, with each patient having his or her own circuit which relates to individual physical ability.

The games section introduces competition. Team games, involving a ball or beanbag, which allow patients to sit or stand depending on their individual physical ability, should be used. A few patients may progress to table tennis in pairs or singles, e.g. a one-game set with the points reduced from the normal scoring system. New patients joining this session will join for shorter periods of time – time being used once more as a grading tool. The old wives' tale 'don't raise your arms above your head' will be dispelled during this session as this action will be required during the ball- or beanbag-catching activity. The therapist gives permission for activity and allows the patient to do the monitoring (pulse recording).

Functional activities

The return of even more independence occurs in the functional activity section of this programme. Monitoring during this section is visual and patients should be expected to recognize personal symptoms if they occur, taking appropriate action by resting or telling the therapist. In this section of the programme the objective is to simulate work (Fig. 4.1b), home or leisure situations. Therapists are present, usually to monitor and guide. The occupational therapist should guide the selection of activity, presenting the patient with a choice. Grading of activity is made by position of work and, as during the exercise session, time and resistance. It is a task-oriented session and each individual works at his or her own pace. Competition will evolve from speed of completion, quality of finished product, design and style, depending on the activity. The selection of task should allow the individual's dexterity, creative ability or other personal attributes to be used and demonstrated. There should be a meaningful end-product.

Activities familiar to an individual should initially be avoided. Low concentration spans have been observed in patients, leading to reduced performance of known tasks. New or unusual activities (to the patient) should therefore be available. Printing or stool-seating are both activities where the position may be upgraded and resistance increased as the activity progresses, and are therefore suitable for use early in the programme. Progress to wood or metal work activities provides suitable activity towards the end of a programme.

It is during the activities section of the programme that the domestic activities causing anxiety may be practised. Kitchen areas may be used for meal preparation, and patients encouraged to make their own coffee, wash up and clear away. Gardening activities may also be introduced if the facilities are available. Job simulation may also be possible depending on the facilities available in the treatment environment – desk activities, sorting, store-keeping or heavy lifting.

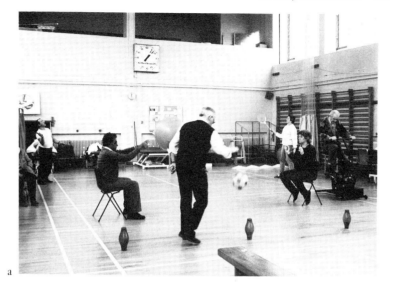

a

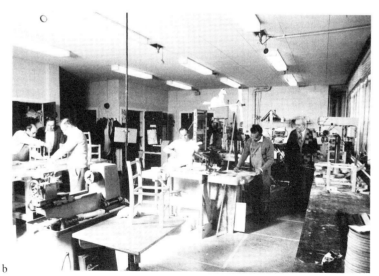

b

Fig. 4.1a, b Regaining confidence through graded physical activities in (a) gymnasium and (b) heavy workshop, as part of an outpatient coronary rehabilitation programme

Both the physiotherapist and occupational therapist need to make use of their assessment skills in identifying individual levels of function. Their skill of activity and exercise analysis is equally important. Depending on the extent of infarction and pre-morbid fitness, each patient will have a different level of tolerance. The selection of activities (or exercise) may superficially appear the same to patients, but the manner of performing the task (or exercise) needs to match the patient's psychological requirement and physical ability. Thus a patient with low physical tolerance may work alongside another in woodwork. The first patient gets a morale boost by using a coping saw, sanding and painting, while the other may use a rip saw or bench plane.

Discharge from an intensive programme such as that described above should be about 4–5 weeks after commencement. The period may be extended for patients with either medical or work complications. During the programme symptoms not identified during hospitalization may develop during or as a result of activity. It is essential that medical staff should be available if required by the therapist and that a response is guaranteed.

Patients are discharged from the programme after they have bargained and reached the stage of acceptance, regained self-confidence and can identify their individual limitations. For patients returning to work the first day may be traumatic. Colleagues all come to say hello and welcome back. Patients should be advised to dispense with the social aspects of the return to work a few days before their official day of return to work, when they can control the length of stay and time of day of the visit.

SELECTION OF PATIENT AND CONCLUSIONS

Given the number of individuals with coronary artery disease it is impossible to organize programmes as described for all patients. It is not possible as yet to identify specifically those patients most at risk of developing handicap following myocardial infarction. The restrictions to quality of life, work and employment potential, in the absence of a rehabilitation programme. identify an at risk population – those of working age – in terms of quality of life. The majority of patients in this age group are male. Within an average health authority (250 000 population) it should be possible to provide a programme for this population with three fulltime therapists, medical back-up facilities and accommodation. This is comparatively inexpensive when compared to the effect rehabilitation can have on the quality of life of not only the patients but also their families.

The economic consequences of rapid rehabilitation and return to work are enormous but have not yet been quantified. An active rehabilitation course is bound to have an impact on reducing the incidence of risk factors for rein-farction and encouraging previously sedentary patients to resume an active and worthwhile life. The opportunity for dietary advice and reduction of serum cholesterol is also bound to have a significant impact and the active rehabilitation period can only be looked upon as essential following myocardial infarction. It is yet to be proven that physical exercise reduces the incidence of further reinfarction but a large number of such trials have been attempted worldwide and all show a positive trend over a 5-year period. Not one of these trials has yet reached statistical significance but each has a trend and there can be no reasonable doubt that the increased muscle tone induced by an active physical rehabilitation programme is beneficial and economically useful.

REFERENCES

1. World Health Organization (1971), *Rehabilitation Programmes for patients with myocardial infarction*, Euro 8206 (6).
2. World Health Organization (1969), *Psychological aspects of the rehabilitation of cardiovascular patients*, Euro 5030.

FURTHER READING

Bilodeau C. B., Hackett, T. P. (1971), Issues raised in a group setting by patients recovering from myocardial infarction, *Am. J. Psychiatry*; **128**: 73–8.

Chatterjee D. S., Parkes H. G. eds. (1982), *Cardiac Rehabilitation – Proceedings of a Society of Occupational Medicine Research Panel Symposium* London, Society of Occupational Medicine.

Dhooper S. S. (1983), Family coping with the crisis of heart attack, *Soc. Work Health Care*; 9: 15–31.

Mann S., Yates J. E., Raftery E. B. (1981), The effect of myocardial infarction on sexual activity, *J. Cardiac Rehab.*; 1: 187–92.

Mayou R. (1984), Prediction of emotional and social outcome after a heart attack, *J. Psychosom. Res.*; **28**: 17–25.

McKendry M., Logan R. L. (1982), The recognition and management of denial in patients after myocardial infarction, *Aust. N.Z. J. Med.*; **12**: 607–11.

Schlesinger Z., Segev U. (1982), Rehabilitation of patients after acute myocardial infarction, *Adv. Cardiol.*; **31**: 226–31.

Sjogren K., Fugl-Meyer A. R. (1983), Some factors influencing sexual life after myocardial infarction, *Int. Rehab. Med.*; 5: 197–201.

Soloff P. H. (1977), Denial and rehabilitation of the post infarction patient. *Int. J. Psychiatr. Med.*; 8: 125–32.

Stockmeier U. ed. (1976), *Psychological Approach to the Rehabilitation of Coronary Patients*. Berlin, Springer Verlag.

van Dixhoorn J. et al (1983), Contribution of relaxation technique training to the re-habilitation of myocardial infarction patients, *Psychother. Psychosom.*; **40**; 137–47.

Walbroehl G. S. (1984), Sexual activity and the post coronary patient, *Am. Fam. Physician*; **29**: 175–7.

Watson P. A. et al (1986), Employment after myocardial infarction amongst pre-viously healthy men, *J. Roy. Soc. Med.*; **79**: 329–30.

5

Stroke

---

with particular reference to the younger patient

Andrew Frank and Sandy Homewood

INTRODUCTION

Stroke is the commonest condition in this country which leads to very severe
disability and thus provides a model for the description of the help needed
by individuals who suffer from a disabling condition, and who have an
expectation of some recovery. The broader problems discussed will be similar to those faced by anyone with acute brain damage. This pattern is in dis-
tinction to patients with multiple sclerosis (who may expect a variable and
uncertain course; (Chapter 8) and those with rapidly progressive conditions
such as motor neurone disease.

The sudden and unexpected onset of a stroke can be devastating. Previously active, confident and self-reliant individuals can lose control over
many aspects of their lives: 'Chained by a disabled body, one feels worthless,
vulnerable and defenceless'.[1] The most immediate loss is likely to be that of
mobility, with the need to become dependent on others for physical functioning, and the resultant humiliation this may cause. Communication difficulties may prevent individuals initiating a conversation or responding to a
question and thus being unable to influence people around them. Social factors such as loss of employment and loss of earnings can lead to a shattering
of ambitions and a loss of self-respect, both within and outside the family.

This chapter will not concentrate on the acute stage in hospital, except to
illustrate how good early care can improve the ultimate outcome. The main
emphasis of the chapter is to consider the process of returning the individual
to as near a normal life as is possible, and will be described in two phases –
physical rehabilitation and social rehabilitation, although both are inter-
related. The final part of this chapter outlines the longer-term consequences
of the stroke.

Both authors primarily have experience with younger stroke patients. The same principles apply in all age groups, but elderly patients are more likely to have multiple impairments, and may be managed by departments of geriatric medicine (see Chapter 7).

EPIDEMIOLOGY

The annual incidence is approximately 2 strokes per 1000 population, which is equivalent to 500 strokes per average health district of 250 000 and 20 per average group practice list of 10 000. It can be assumed, however, that one-third will die before leaving hospital, and rather less than one-third will have a total recovery. Thus less than a half will remain as disabled stroke survivors. Each family doctor may therefore look after approximately two new disabled stroke victims per year. There have been few good studies on the prevalence of stroke-induced disability, but in one study only one-third of the stroke victims survived for 1 year.[2] A higher incidence among males than females over the age of 54 is commonly observed, and in the same study, three-quarters of the stroke victims were older than 69.[2] The epidemiology is well reviewed elsewhere (see further reading).

CARE AT HOME

There are no good data related to the extent of hospitalization after stroke, but it would appear that at least one-third of all stroke victims are managed at home by their general practitioners. The individual may have mild symptoms such that a crisis admission is not indicated, may refuse to go into hospital, there may be no hospital bed available, or the individual may be clearly dying, and the family may wish to provide terminal care at home.

The brunt of providing care will be taken by relatives, helped by friends and neighbours. The general practitioner aims to co-ordinate the resources of the district nursing service, domiciliary physiotherapy and community-based occupational therapists, and must be aware of additional local services that will help to support the family – everything from domiciliary chiropody to financial help and allowances may be requested by relatives seeking support. The district nurse is often the most closely involved and will assess the needs of the individual and teach the relatives how to care for the patient between her visits. The stroke patient's blood pressure should be checked as it tends to fluctuate after a stroke, and particularly in the elderly, incontinence, infection and skin breakdown may be present. The number of visits will vary depending on the severity of the stroke and the ability of the relatives. The emotional state of all family members must be monitored.

The community occupational therapist will advise on increasing personal independence and will provide necessary adaptations and equipment to facilitate this. Relatives should be encouraged to promote increased activity and independence and assist the individual in returning to his or her former recreations and social life. The correct balance must be sought to avoid sacrificing the quality of the relatives' lives for the sake of the individual. General practitioners can gauge this balance in view of their likely previous knowledge of the family. Where domiciliary physiotherapists are not available the district nurse and general practitioner will introduce a rehabilitation programme. Frequently, this is facilitated by attending the district general hospital stroke rehabilitation programme, local day centre, or geriatric day hospital.

The majority of individuals will, however, be admitted to hospital, and the remainder of the chapter describes hospital-oriented practice, though most of the principles are identical whether a patient is treated at home or in hospital.

THE ACUTE STAGE

In the few days following admission, the main focus of the relatives and the individual will be the risk of dying. The uncertainty created may lead to false expectations once recovery is assured, resulting in disillusion and despair when the extent of ultimate disability is revealed. The medical problems are outside the scope of this chapter, but cover the exclusion of brain tumour or heart disease as causes of the stroke and sometimes the differentiation of an ischaemic stroke from a haemorrhagic stroke.

General management aims to prevent pressure sores, limb contractures, hypostatic pneumonia and loss of morale. Nursing care given in the early stages is not only supportive and preventative but essential to future rehabilitation. Whether conscious or unconscious, patients are regarded as individuals who have suffered a stroke. When the patients are comatose it is important that nurses should always talk to them during nursing care as if they were awake. A continuous drip feed, usually via a nasogastric tube, provides sufficient energy for the body needs. The physiotherapist will give chest physiotherapy to prevent the accumulation of secretions and will perform passive movements in functional movement patterns. When spasticity develops, positioning of the limbs needs to be in reflex-inhibiting positions, thus necessitating close collaboration between the physiotherapists and the nursing staff. Care needs to be taken to avoid trauma to the shoulder of the hemiplegic arm, particularly when it is flaccid, especially when turning patients, sitting them up in bed or assisting in transferring. Urinary incontinence may require temporary catheterization or the use of condom drainage in men (see Chapter 6) and a stool softener may be required to prevent constipation.

On recovery of consciousness, patients are encouraged to do as much for themselves as possible with the additional help of rehabilitation staff, who should encourage activities with an emphasis on the affected side. Such activities help counteract the 'neglect' of the affected side often shown by individuals with sensory and perceptual disturbances. Individuals with brain stem involvement may require close collaboration between the speech therapist, dietitian and nurse (see below).

During the acute stage it is often the ward sister who plays a co-ordinating role, who sees the spouse and/or relatives and who may first notice the implications of the stroke for the family. She may arrange for a social worker to see the individual or spouse if this has not already taken place. At this stage the family is usually too distressed to participate in counselling, but the offer of future help and the ability to listen to fraught relatives may be extremely important. Explanation of the need for medical, nursing and rehabilitative procedures or treatments also contributes to their participation and ability to cope with the situation, both emotionally and practically.

Optimum recovery may be dependent on the motivation of the individual. Sympathetic nursing during the acute phase contributes greatly to the essential preservation of the individual's self-respect.

PHYSICAL REHABILITATION

The initial major objective is to enable the individual to become personally independent. The important areas lie in communication, mobility, transfers (in and out of bed, on and off chairs and toilet), washing and dressing. Particular help is necessary for patients with difficulties in communication as both families and specialist staff find this impairment a major cause of distress and demoralization.

It is the development of multiprofessional team work which is likely to be one of the key factors in the success of stroke wards.[3] Such team work is fostered by weekly meetings of all staff to assess progress and co-ordinate activities which encourage the patient to become more independent. Another attribute likely to be effective in increasing patients' independence and decreasing hospital length of stay is the early concentration on the social aspects of care. Involvement of families in the rehabilitation of loved ones may help to reduce the risk of over-protection which can destroy the individual's potential for independence. Similarly, early assessment of possible family or environmental problems which will be faced at discharge is helpful.

Communication, nutrition and feeding

When patients have communication difficulties, early assessment by a speech therapist is essential. This gives confidence to patients and relatives and may assist staff in communicating with the patient. Where there is a pure dysarthria, simple communication aids may facilitate early communication. The detailed management of dysphasia is outside the scope of this chapter. Stress, euphoria, confusion, hearing loss, fatigue and the effects of medication may all impede communication. When comatose patients become conscious, speech therapists may advise on the timing of withdrawal of the nasogastric tube. Dysphagia is common after a severe stroke and often patients manage soft foods better than liquids alone and can still receive a balanced diet, thus avoiding a gain in weight. Feeding gives another example of team work, where the dietitian, occupational and speech therapists, and nurses plan to overcome the difficulties in feeding. Patients are encouraged to feed themselves but many initially complicated tasks such as cutting certain foods, spreading butter etc. may require help, as may feeding itself. Simple aids may facilitate eating and drinking (Table 5.1) and greatly reduce the indignity consequent upon being fed.

Where drinking is difficult, poor fluid intake (perhaps compounded by immobility) may lead to constipation. This may require more bulk, initially puréed vegetables and fruit, and later wholemeal bread, cereals or bran.

It is always important to involve the patient in the choice of foods on the menu, and in relating these choices to food texture.

Working towards independence

The initial objective is to maximize mobility, and this is usually supervised by physiotherapists. The physiotherapist concentrates on the following problems: 'neglect' and 'loss of body image' resulting from sensory and perceptual disturbances (Fig. 5.1); alteration of muscle tone resulting in flaccidity or spasticity; partial or complete loss of voluntary control of the affected side; and forgotten 'normal' movement patterns. In spite of extensive physiotherapy, walking aids may be required, as may orthoses to prevent

Table 5.1   An indication of the extent of available equipment

Activity	Equipment
Washing	
Standing balance	High stool
Bathing	
Standing balance	High stool
Access (ambulant)	Bath board, bath seat, bath mat, rail
Access (semi- and non-ambulant)	Swivel, adjustable height chair hoist
	Bath seat raised/lowered by air/water pressure
	Mobile hoist with sling
Reach for washing	Long-handled sponge/brush
	Rubber hose
Securing items	Suction nailbrush
	Soap inside flannel mitt
Toilet	
Getting on and off	Toilet frame fixed to floor/rails
	Raised toilet seat
Mobility difficulties	Commode sited by bed
	Chemical toilet sited downstairs
Dressing	
Reaching	Dressing stick
Reaching/lack of balance	Long-handled pick-up stick
Manipulation	Large hooks, sticks, velcro to replace buttons, slip-on tie, front-fastening bra, elastic shoelaces, rings/tags
Bed	
General assistance	Lifting pole and stand, rails fixed to wall or bed, portable or fixed hoist
Getting on and off	Bed blocks, or bed-raising units
	Boards under mattress to firm it
Turning	Boards under mattress to firm it
Sitting up	Rope ladder
Chair	
Getting in and out	Chair blocks or chair-raising unit
Poor posture	High seat/high-back upright armchair
Eating/drinking	
Weak grip in affected hand	Enlarged handled/angled cutlery, cups
Cutting food	Rocker knife

Table 5.1   *continued*

Activity	Equipment
Eating/drinking *continued*	
Cutting/eating same hand	Combined knife/fork, or knife/fork/spoon
Securing food on plate	Plate with raised concave edge
	Plate with guard attached to edge of plate
Securing implement on table	Non-slip mat
	Suction base
Keeping food hot	Hot water compartment under dish
Kitchen	
Carrying items	Trolley
	Non-slip one-handled tray
Balance	High stool
Stabilizing	Non-slip mat, suction bases, clamps, cut-out in work surface to hold bowl, board with spikes to secure vegetables, board with grater fixed to it, peeler clamped to work surface, bean slicer clamped to work surface, box grater, kettle/teapot tippers
Opening	Wall-mounted/electric can openers, various rubber bottle and jar openers, multigrip scissors
Whisking	One-handled pump action whisk
	Electic whisk
Spreading	Board with two raised edges which are pushed against when spreading
Straining vegetables	Vegetable basket inside saucepan
Cleaning	
Washing floors and windows	Long-handled squeeze mop
Sweeping	Long-handled dustpan and brush
Communication	
Reading	Talking books
Writing	Enlarged/angled handles to writing utensils, paperweight, magnet, dycem to stabilize paper, typewriter
Telephone	GPO headset, loud-speaking or 'no hands' conversation telephone etc., many types available
Expression	Charts, mechanical and electronic equipment (supplied under supervision of a speech therapist)

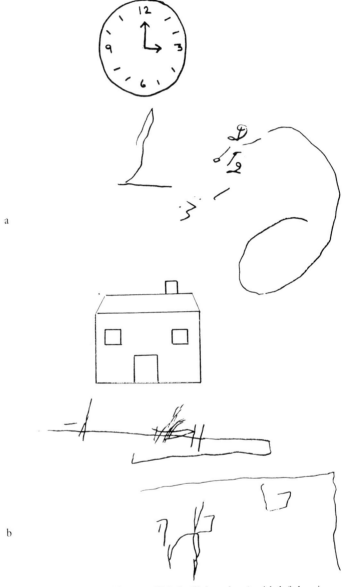

Fig. 5.1a, b   Drawings of an 81-year-old lady (living alone) with left hemiplegia, no sensory problems, no dysphasia, but loss of midline orientation. Figures depict an inability to centralize pictures and demonstrate additional visual spacial problems aggravated by fatigue. Such deficits are often not apparent during routine enquiry but explain her inability to stand unaided

foot drop. We believe patients should understand from an early stage that physiotherapy maximizes the return of function allowed by the restoration of brain function during recovery. It should not be considered to be curative. To encourage this idea is to lead patients to expect on-going treatment even after their condition plateaus, and also to continue to deny the unacceptable prospect of prolonged disablement when their physiotherapy is gradually withdrawn. At this stage the occupational therapist will work towards the restoration of everyday skills (e.g. washing and dressing; Fig. 5.2) and will work with others to improve transfers. Motivation and consequently morale improve when physical treatment is integrated into the achievement of independence-oriented objectives.

A few patients have severe cognitive impairment which may limit attempts of family, friends and professionals to help them. Early evaluation by a clinical psychologist may help to define these areas of impairment and serial assessments will identify the rate of improvement. Occasionally behavioural modification techniques may help management early, as well as later on in the recovery process. Thalamic pain may also hinder all attempts at rehabilitation, and in these cases carbamazepine (Tegretol) may be helpful.

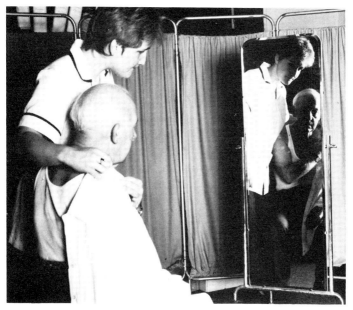

Fig. 5.2 Use of mirror to surmount difficulties in dressing caused by unilateral neglect following cerebrovascular accident

Confidence and social interaction

Confidence returns as progress towards independence is achieved. All staff should encourage communication and social interaction in everyday situations, and specific activities in the occupational therapy hospital workshops are designed to enhance good positioning and awareness of the affected limbs. For patients with milder strokes, a return to previous work-type or leisure activities is encouraged. More severely affected individuals, however, may need to develop new and different activities and interests. A 'ward hostess' has helped social interaction,[4] and relatives' groups have been useful in Bristol, similar to groups used in coronary rehabilitation (see pp. 103, 106).

Early emotional and social consequences

Once the acute stage has passed, the fear of death or loss of a loved one is overtaken by practical and emotional problems. Four stages of adjustment to stroke have been identified (Table 5.2). In the first few weeks, whilst the recovery rate is at its greatest, both patient and carers may have high expectations for recovery. The possibility of permanent disability may be denied.

Table 5.2   Reaction of families to stroke[5]

First stage: crisis
Shock
Confusion
High anxiety

Second stage: treatment
High expectations of recovery
Denial that disability is permanent
Periods of grieving
Fears for future
  Job
  Mobility
  Lifestyle
  About coping

Third stage: realization of disability
Anger
Feelings of rejection
Despair
Frustration
Depression

Final stage: adjustment

Practical problems usually focus around finance, housing and employment. Emotional problems relate to role change, the marital relationship, the effect on the children and the extended family and the emotional and health problems of the spouse. These problems may surface in hospital or develop during or as a consequence of the home visits when it is realized that the individual returning home may not be the same person as he or she was before the stroke.

As therapists spend much time with the patient during this period they help the adjustment process by talking about the disability and discouraging false hopes whilst maintaining enthusiasm. Family members should be encouraged to meet therapists regularly to discuss progress and adjustment.

The social worker, apart from assisting with practical difficulties (e.g. financial), offers counselling to the patient and spouse. This is especially necessary if there is a significant reversal of roles (see Fig. 5.3). One important aspect to be considered is whether a working spouse will continue in employment once his or her potentially dependent partner is discharged home. Often the caring agencies can provide adequate support during weekdays to enable employment to continue. The patient may attend rehabilitation programmes within hospitals, younger disabled units, or day centres. Alternatively, or in addition, monitoring at home may be provided by a team of community-based workers.

The home visit and planning discharge from hospital

Within a few weeks of admission, it is clear whether patients should expect severe residual disability. If so, they may be discharged from hospital when they and their families can cope, and not when they have achieved their optimal potential. In this situation, the home visit is an important step in their rehabilitation.

Once the discharge appears feasible, a conference should be convened where the professional staff from the hospital meet representatives of the community nursing and social services to plan further rehabilitation. The social service representatives will usually include the patient's social worker, a domiciliary occupational therapist, a representative from the day centre, the organizer of the home-help service, and a representative of any scheme locally designed to support the main carer (see Chapter 13). The social services department will usually designate a key worker to co-ordinate the different responsibilities supplied by its department. Hospital members will include representatives of the medical staff, ward sister, and the therapist(s) involved in treating the patient. A general practitioner usually has pertinent information about the physical and emotional health of the family which is invaluable. There are often difficulties in convening meetings between hospital staff and general practitioners, but the district nurse may act as a representative of the general practitioner. The social worker may bring the patient and/or spouse for part or all of the conference. This ensures that all aspects of the situation are discussed and the wishes of the patient and family are clearly expressed.

The conference will usually plan an initial home visit of the patient and the occupational therapist(s), who will be responsible for supplying equipment or advising on adaptations to the home. A provisional date of discharge is planned. On rare occasions, it may be decided that the person cannot be supported in the community, in which event placement in health or social service residential accommodation will be considered.

The home visit aims to predetermine the practical difficulties likely to be faced after discharge. It will determine the suitability of the site of the bedroom and toilets, and often will result in a bed being moved downstairs for short-term use, and in the provision of a downstairs commode. Difficulties with steps or slopes (inside or outside the home) are identified and plans made to overcome them with ramps and rails if needed (Table 5.3).

Having arranged these basic adaptations, the patient can spend a 24-hour period at home. This may be prudently arranged midweek, when nursing and other support are more easily provided. Following this trial visit, both patient and spouse can discuss with staff the real or imagined difficulties, and plans can be made to overcome them.

A trial period at home also identifies likely difficulties in terms of the

Table 5.3 Adaptations commonly supplied for hemiplegic people

Difficulty	Ambulant	Chairbound
Access to property	Shallow steps, extra rails	Ramp
Doorways	Doors re-hung	Widened
Stairs	Handrails	Stairlift Elevator
Sockets	Raised	Raised
Bathroom and toilet	Rails by bath and toilet	Ground floor extension Shower instead of bath
Kitchen	Re-positioning of storage and work areas	Convert to wheelchair kitchen
Mobility	Door-opening intercom Personal alarm	Door-opening intercom Personal alarm

carer's reaction to the return home and the couple's coping ability. For many families the discharge from hospital is seen as the vital objective. In reality discharge is the beginning of a life of adjustment to disability which is so complex that initially a reactive depression is common. Home visits have an important role to play in beginning the adjustment before leaving hospital.

Provided good outpatient rehabilitation facilities exist, discharge can proceed as soon as practical on a pre-arranged date.

Major adaptations will often take place after discharge. This may reflect the time involved in instigating such work. At the time of discharge the degree of recovery from the stroke cannot always be predicted. It is therefore sensible to delay the commencement of a potentially large and expensive adaptation until further needs can be accurately established. At the time of the return home, many individuals and their families may still have unrealistically high expectations of recovery (Table 5.2; second stage) and are psychologically not ready to accept permanent alterations to their home.

Local authority occupational therapists are aware of these limiting factors and take them into account when advising the best type of adaptation to suit the situation. They will also liaise with the architect, surveyor and builder, and support the individual and family until completion.

If the property is privately owned and lends itself to the appropriate alterations, government improvement grants are available, which, in conjunction with financial help also given by many local authorities, will usually cover the majority of costs involved.

Voluntary housing associations also provide specially designed housing, and for those who cannot manage to live alone there are private and local authority-run sheltered housing blocks. However, for the younger individual, these are hard to find.

Aids and/or equipment for independent living

Functional difficulties experienced will differ according to the varied results of a stroke. The level of mobility will depend not only on the amount of recovery from paralysis, but also on the degree of spasticity, sensory loss and cerebellar involvement.

If perceptual problems occur (usually in right hemisphere lesions), difficulties with body shape and its position in space will affect mobility, and associated lack of 'body image' will make many activities, like dressing, extremely difficult. Often these difficulties can be overcome with training and the use of compensatory techniques. Thus, patients can be taught to check visually the position of a limb, or, in the case of hemianopia, to turn the head to the affected side as much as possible to increase the range of vision. Commonly the individual will need to learn one-handed methods which will be more difficult with the non-dominant hand. All new learning techniques can be hampered by lack of concentration, difficulties with remembering, acquired communication problems, and by the tendency to tire quickly. Breaking down activities into easy stages with regular, short training sessions and plenty of encouragement in an environment that is without distractions is usually the most successful way to assist in the learning process.

Expressive and receptive communication difficulties require careful and detailed assessment. Initially they may be helped by the use of gesture, picture cards, or simple written material. Communication aids may be useful for a small number of individuals with motor defects.

There are many aids available to assist functioning (Table 5.1). It is always desirable to attempt the many varied alternative methods and techniques in carrying out an activity before an aid is supplied, but if an aid improves function without the need to rely on another person then it is increasing that individual's independence and its use should be encouraged. This subject is extensively reviewed in *Help Yourselves*,[6] and where rehabilitation takes place without advice from rehabilitation staff, this book can be recommended to stroke victims and their families.

SOCIAL REHABILITATION

Whilst the social consequences of the stroke have been stressed from the beginning of this chapter (see section on the acute stage, above) and play their part throughout the period of physical rehabilitation, we believe that insufficient thought has been given, particularly by hospital-based programmes, to the technical aspects of restoring individuals to the best quality of life attainable. Hence the term 'social rehabilitation' which complements physical rehabilitation initially, but then becomes the main objective of management. The voluntary sector has flourished in this area due possibly to professional neglect (see p. 235). This section of the chapter starts with the outpatient still receiving intensive hospital-based rehabilitation.

Outpatient management

Hospital discharge will often precede the cessation of physical recovery, and rehabilitation will continue on an outpatient basis. It has been shown that the degree of independence achieved is influenced by the amount of outpatient rehabilitation given. Four visits to the outpatient clinic weekly are of most value, but in practice few departments are able to provide this. In

Harrow this may be combined with social rehabilitation at the local social services day centre (see below).

The lack of satisfactory ambulance services may limit the effectiveness of outpatient rehabilitation. The voluntary car service is often unable to cope with the demands made on it. In rural areas the problem may be solved by the use of hostel-type accommodation.

When the rate of physical improvement decreases, a transitional period commences when people are gradually weaned away from physical therapy. This cessation of physical treatment finally seals in the minds of the 'stroke family' the degree of permanent disability which is likely to result. A physiotherapy 'at risk register' reassures all concerned that further advice can be given if needed. In Harrow we are fortunate in having a day centre (see below) for younger people with disabilities which is able to help at this stage. We find it helpful to tell patients that, whilst their physical rehabilitation is drawing to a close, their social rehabilitation is just beginning. Speech therapy may continue for months or years and communication skills are further encouraged at the day centre.

Where the individual has a working spouse or carer, it is our policy to help the spouse to continue at work if at all possible. Thus the spouse has links with the 'real world' whilst the family world disintegrates and then re-integrates. Consequently, it may be arranged for individuals to attend the day centre immediately after discharge on those days when there is no hospital-based rehabilitation. This programme is arranged at the pre-discharge case conference (see p. 123).

Role of the day centre

Many areas have day centres for handicapped individuals of working age, and their potential objectives are listed in Table 5.4. Such centres may be

Table 5.4 Potential objectives of day centres for the hemiplegic person

Continue physical rehabilitation

Assist social reintegration – relationships with others

Assist transition from old lifestyle to new

Rehabilitate into employment and/or develop new interests

Support carers and share responsibility for care

Relieve individual and/or carer of excessive company of each other organized by health services (sometimes as a younger disabled unit), the voluntary sector, or social services, or any combination.

Day centres are usually in a non-medical setting which encourages handicapped individuals to reorientate themselves away from a 'patient' self-image to that of a self-reliant person. Individuals are encouraged to take an equal part in decision-making about present and future participation in a community style environment.

A contract may be made between the attender and the centre in which common aims are set out and this contract should be reviewed and updated regularly. There needs to be continuous liaison with the fieldworker from social services and the hospital remedial staff to ensure that what is happening at home and in outpatient rehabilitation can be paralleled or contrasted at the centre. The day centre will probably employ occupational therapists who provide the link between physical and social rehabilitation. The activities may vary according to staff input and individual or group needs.

From the commencement of attendance it is necessary for the individual and family to realize that the day centre resources are to be used as a stepping stone towards reintegration into society. It will be detrimental for a long-term dependence to be formed, as can easily happen in a safe and protected environment, especially where other attenders with deteriorating conditions require varying amounts of care.

From the outset there is an expectation of active participation by the individual in decision-making as well as in all practical activities with an understanding that this participation will take place increasingly outside the centre. To facilitate this the centre should ideally be situated close to local community resources and there should be access to public and specialist transport. The day centre building should look as normal as possible. If its use by other members of the public is encouraged this has the added benefit of helping society to understand and accept the disability of those who attend.

The role a day centre can play is illustrated by a civil servant, aged 50, married with two teenage children, who suffered an intracerebral haemorrhage resulting in a right hemiplegia and dysphasia. At discharge from hospital he was able to walk unaided for 100 metres, had a functionless right arm and a severe expressive dysphasia with mild receptive loss. His programme is outlined in Table 5.5.

Support groups

Support groups for carers and relatives can do much to alleviate some of the frustration and anxiety felt in caring for a stroke sufferer. Where there is

Table 5.5 Illustrative day centre programme of social rehabilitation

Tasks	Liaison person(s)
Early stages	
Walking practice – indoors and outdoors	Hospital physiotherapist
Standing tolerance	
Personal functioning – dressing, bathing, kitchen activities	Community occupational therapist re: bathroom alterations Hospital occupational therapist
Physical skills – function of non-dominant hand, standing tolerance in pottery, art, light woodwork	Hospital occupational therapist
Social reintegration, i.e. drama group, reinstating old hobbies, instigating new ones	Hospital occupational therapist and hospital social worker
Communication – reading, writing and speech, typing, figure work	Hospital speech therapist

Objective	Liaison person(s)
Later stages (transition from physical to social rehabilitation increased)	
Expand interests and hobbies, i.e. furniture restoration, computing, pottery, horticulture, keep-fit, social outings, local education classes	Social worker
Improve task-sharing at home. Shopping, kitchen activities, household budgeting and finances	Community occupational therapist
Practice leisure activities (acquired or performed in day centre) at home and in the community	Other centre staff
Improve self-reliance: camping holidays, Jubilee Sailing Trust (Chapter 14)	

communication loss, the emotional strain on the spouse is generally that much greater. Much mutual support can be gained by carers who share common problems and discuss new ways of coping.

Frequently carers have been unable to assimilate all the information given to them in the earlier stages by various hospital and social services personnel and a support group can assist the process of assimilation by inviting various speakers to discuss their roles in the rehabilitation process. A support group may be run formally with professional input to provide information and facilitate discussion; it may be an informal mutual support group with no professional input, a combination of both styles or organised by a branch of the Association of Carers (Chapter 14).

For those carers on whom the stroke sufferer is totally dependent, a 'sitting' service may enable them to attend the group (Chapter 13).

The voluntary sector

Some areas have Stroke Groups which provide a strong social component. These have all the attributes of self-help groups (Chapter 13), but have the extra advantage of giving practice in communication. They may be hospital-based, run by social services, or perhaps more commonly by local volunteers through the Chest, Heart and Stroke Association (see Chapter 14). In some areas, this association also supports volunteer schemes whereby individuals are visited at home and assisted with communication, memory and perceptual difficulties, in association with the local speech therapy service. The Chest, Heart and Stroke Association has informative leaflets which may be helpful (see Chapter 14).

Voluntary groups can also assist in other ways including transportation (i.e. voluntary car pool attached to the local hospital, community transport schemes etc.) This is particularly important when one considers that socially oriented rehabilitation may be a low priority in an overworked ambulance service. In our area, a hospital-based Stroke Club ceased to function largely due to transport difficulties. Other groups help with practical needs, e.g. decorating and gardening.

The voluntary services which have developed in relation to patients discharged from the Bristol Stroke Unit include individual and group help to meet many needs. There a group exists for men of working age to share common interests; likewise, a ladies' group, skittles groups and a garden for the disabled.[5]

The voluntary sector can also help certain individuals who find professionally organized social programmes unacceptable; however, there are still many individuals who do not wish to join groups, or who feel patronized by the offer of voluntary services.[5]

Longer-term adjustment

Some families adjust to the problems created by a member having a stroke better than others (Table 5.2; third stage). Much depends on the interrelationships within the family prior to the stroke, and the type of role each family member has played. Almost all families find that however close or self-contained the relationships, and however dominant or submissive the roles, an occurrence so sudden and unexpected as a stroke will cause anxiety and bewilderment which may persist for years. Counselling tries to assist individuals and their families in coming to terms with the situation. When it is clear that a family is having profound difficulties at adjustment, there should be agreement by all involved as to who will do the counselling. Usually social workers are most likely to combine the counselling skills with the time needed to give to the family. However, care needs to be taken to ensure close collaboration with the other caring professionals in order that a common approach may be maintained.

Recent studies have inferred that the adjustment that has to take place following discharge is harder than anticipated. The transition period from hospital to home is critical as both patient and family realize that the progress gained in hospital still leaves much to be desired in the context of family and community living. This stage resembles a state of bereavement. Wage-earners may realize that they can no longer be the 'provider' in financial and perhaps in emotional terms. Lack of physical progress, loneliness and a change in lifestyle may result in frustration, loss of confidence and loss of concentration. Feelings of uselessness may develop and depression may result. Constant encouragement is needed to talk about these feelings and help to identify roles in the family that can be fulfilled. Many of these roles may be new and encouragement will be required to help the individual to participate and interact. This process is complicated where there is dysphasia or intellectual impairment, in particular loss of memory. Other family members share a sense of loss. The subsequent tension may result in tiredness and fatigue, particularly in a spouse. Many find that the effort of keeping the family functioning is very stressful, particularly in the context of the fear of a possible future stroke. The spouse may feel that the partner is not trying hard enough, or feel guilty that in some way he or she 'caused' the stroke to happen.

Figure 5.3 shows some reactions to a stroke which may be found in extreme situations. A dominant partner may have difficulty in allowing the spouse to fight to regain independence, and may be unable to see the importance of the time-consuming struggle, day after day, to get dressed. How much easier and quicker it is to do it for the partner! This, however, will reduce even further any future independence the individual may develop. At the other extreme, the spouse may not cope. The extra responsibilities become too great. Ill health may result, taking a number of forms – depression, backache, alcohol abuse or road traffic accidents. The general

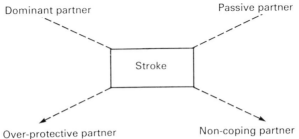

Fig. 5.3   Possible outcomes for a relationship interrupted by stroke

practitioner is best equipped to be aware of partners at risk in this situation and to maximize the help available in the hope of maintaining the health of the spouse, and thus the viability of the relationship.

The sexual side of a relationship may suffer, and feelings of revulsion and/or self-revulsion may be helped with counselling. Practical advice regarding positioning and techniques may be helpful. The fear of a further stroke, which may be out of proportion, may inhibit one or both partners from further sexual activity. 'Stroke families' do not always find it easy to get appropriate advice.

Once the family has faced its interpersonal losses, the process of longer-term adjustment (Table 5.2; final stage) can be assisted by aiming to fulfil new and complementary roles. The individual must have the opportunity to contribute positively to family life and to develop meaningful activities. These may include local interest groups or courses on a wide variety of subjects run by the local College of Education. Hobbies or recreational activities, both familiar and new, can be taken up, and some of these are listed in Table 5.6.

Employment

Many hemiplegic people benefit from help in returning to work, though if their original employment proves unsuitable the present economic climate makes alternatives difficult to find. Generally an office job is easier to return to than a manual one. The Employment Services Section of the Training Commission formerly the Manpower Services Commission is empowered to arrange adaptations and alterations to the working environment to suit the individual's needs. A former employer may be sympathetic in finding an alternative type of job within the company which is more suited to the needs of the disabled person.

The Disablement Resettlement Officer (DRO) works in the local job

Table 5.6 Some recreational activities that can be adapted for the hemiplegic person

Leisure	Sport and physical recreation
Art	Archery
Board and card games	Bowls
Gardening	Dancing
Knitting	Fishing
Musical instruments	Flying
Photography (Fig. 5.4)	Golf
Pottery	Riding
Printing	Sailing
Sewing	Skiing
Woodwork	Swimming

centre, and is employed by the Training Commission to help disabled people remain in or find employment. The DRO may also recommend alternative training, assessment at an employment rehabilitation centre, or sheltered employment.

Specific assistance can be given by a day centre or rehabilitation department where applicable, which is geared towards improving confidence and the ability of the individual in relation to the type of job, i.e. simulated clerical tasks, use of the telephone, message-taking, the issuing of clear instructions, and operating technical equipment. Confidence can also be developed in practising coping with public transport over the route to and from work. The Training Commission may contribute towards the cost of private transport to and from work.

A trial period at work whilst the individual remains on sickness benefit may help to ensure that the planned return to work is not premature, and that both employer and employee are confident of its success. When returning to work, some flexibility in the timing and duration of the working day helps to avoid unnecessary fatigue caused, for example, by travelling in the rush hour.

Mobility and driving

The combination of physical and cognitive impairment may make a return to driving impossible. All those disabled for more than 3 months following a stroke must declare their disability to the Driver and Vehicle Licensing Centre (DVLC). A recent study has shown that many drivers who were

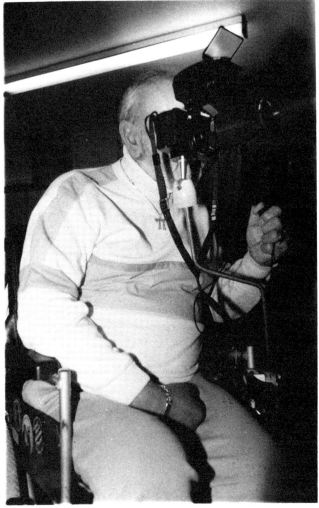

Fig. 5.4 Adapted camera and camera stand attached to wheelchair for a hemiplegic photographer. Reproduced with permission of Graham Hulme

driving prior to their stroke were unable to continue to do so and many of those who do continue have not informed the DVLC.

It is illegal to return to driving if the horizontal visual field is less than 120°. Thus a complete lower quadrantic defect or a homonymous hemi-anopia is a contraindication to driving. Another factor which militates against a return to driving is the time taken from visual perception to the initiation of a driving manoeuvre. This can only be evaluated currently by a driving assessment.[7] Such assessments can be performed in a number of centres (see Appendix 5.1).

Individuals who are unable to drive may suffer increased isolation which may contribute to depression. Consideration needs to be given to the use of outdoor wheelchairs (see Appendix 5.1). Many cars are easily modified and some are specially designed for users of both manual and electric wheel-chairs.

For those whose stroke occurs under the age of 65, the mobility allowance is payable, and may be used in a variety of ways. In many areas there are a wide variety of schemes to help disabled people become more mobile. Such schemes are discussed in Appendix 5.1.

LONG-TERM OUTCOME

This final section considers the long-term outcome, reported elsewhere.[5,8] Although not strictly comparable, these studies show the devastation to the individual and family which may persist for years following a stroke.

Physical dependence

It is likely that the majority of disabled stroke patients are unable to walk outdoors, or only rarely go out. Many will require a walking aid, and a significant number will have to continue sleeping downstairs. In one study 14% still used commodes[5]. In the same study, whilst 70% did not change housing, there were many for whom a change of home would have been desirable, and 15% went into institutional care. In the second study,[8] two-thirds required help in one or more of the following: personal hygiene, feeding, and dressing.

Employment and finances

Less than one-third of individuals in employment prior to their stroke are likely to remain in employment.[8] The chances of employment if there is a persisting hemiplegia are remote. Many individuals reduce their hours of work and change the nature of their work. Approximately one-half of spouses working at the time of the stroke are able to continue working.

The majority of families, therefore, are considerably disadvantaged financially. Many will be eligible for financial assistance from the state (see

Chapter 13), but not everyone claims allowances to which they are entitled. One-half of spouses are likely to worry about the finances.

Health

In the broad sense of the word, few individuals regain full health even though their physical condition stabilizes — the event has been too traumatic. One-third of individuals, and one-third of spouses, are not fully adjusted 2–3 years after the stroke, though not necessarily of the same marriages. Both individual and spouse fear a further stroke not only in the stroke victim, but also in the spouse. Over the period of Holbrook's study, two spouses died of strokes and two of coronaries.[5]

Stroke sufferers are likely to experience many of the following: loss of confidence, inability to concentrate, forgetting intentions and information, mislaying things, feelings of uselessness and loneliness. Two-thirds of spouses will notice personality changes in their partners such as irritability, loss of self-control, impatience, lowered tolerance to frustration, emotional lability, self-centredness and reduced initiative.

Depression and frustration are evident in both patients and spouses, and the depression in the stroke victim may be clinically significant, and yet untreated although treatment is often effective. Tension or depression is less frequent in patients with no previous psychiatric history than in those previously treated. Similarly, tension or depression is more common in spouses with a previous history.[8]

Many spouses have symptoms which reflect an anxiety state and may have been treated with a minor tranquilliser (e.g. a benzodiazepine). This proportion is much higher in spouses of aphasic patients, who are also more lonely, more bored and make a poorer adjustment than spouses of non-aphasic patients. Generally spouses also suffer stress, tiredness, and have difficulties with keeping family harmony and remaining loving.[5]

Marital and sexual relationships

Many of the factors noted above have an effect on the marriage. Loss of communication between partners is likely to be a vital element and has been noted even in the absence of an overt language disorder, perhaps partly arising from the non-handicapped partner's reluctance to bring up emotionally loaded topics. When an individual is dependent on his or her partner for some aspects of daily living, this can cause changing roles in the partnership and in turn shift the emphasis on roles concerning sexuality. Individuals who were sexually active and interested before a stroke may continue to experience sexual interest and desire after a stroke, but most experience a significant decrease in sexual function. Men may note difficulties in erection and ejaculation, and women cessation of menses and lack of orgasm.

Thus, fear of further strokes, particularly during intercourse; disruption of the normal rhythm of married life by illness, and meeting dependent needs; physical aversion towards the disabled partner; depression in either partner and anxiety in the non-disabled partner; and changes in personality all combine to disrupt the marital relationship. Decreased sexual activity is one symptom of this disruption, and may be complicated by side-effects of antihypertensive drugs, amongst others. In spite of this, at least three couples are reported as having their first child following a stroke in one partner.[8] Children are also affected by the stroke in a parent. Apart from the initial shock, the most serious effect may be the relationship of the stroke victim with the child. Personality change, communication difficulties and mobility all affect children. Whilst some children were thought to experience an 'unhappy home life', others 'matured more rapidly'.[8]

CONCLUSIONS

Stroke is used as a model illness to discuss the effects of acute brain damage on individuals and their families. After the initial crisis, a period of physical rehabilitation aimed at the restoration of independence is described. At the same time, rather insidiously, social rehabilitation commences, helping individuals and their families to come to terms with the illness and the awful realization that recovery has led to disability. Some means by which a gradual reintegration into their family and society may be achieved are described.

In spite of apparently good physical and social rehabilitation, the outlook for many is disheartening. Immobility, dependence, difficulty in communication and changes in personality may be present and impede the restoration of stability for the victim and the 'stroke family'. Depression, frustration and minor psychiatric disorders are all frequently seen in stroke survivors and their spouses.

REFERENCES

1. Anker H. (1985), By a stroke of luck, *Br. Med. J.*; **291**: 1792–5.
2. Stevens R. S., Ambler N. R. (1982), The incidence and survival of stroke patients in a defined community, *Age Ageing*; **11**: 266–74.

3. Stephens R. S. (1984), Stroke rehabilitation units in the United Kingdom, *Health Trends*; **16**: 61–3.
4. Isaacs B. (1977), Five years experience of a stroke unit, *Health Bull. Edinburgh*; **35**: 93–8.
5. Holbrook M. (1982), Stroke: social and emotional outcome, *J. Roy. Coll. Phys. (Lond)*; **16**: 100–4.
6. Jay P. E. (1985), *Help Yourselves: A Handbook for Hemiplegics and their Families*, Kincardin, Ian D. Henry Publications.
7. Simms B. (1985), Perception and driving – theory and practice, *Occup. Ther.*; **48**: 363–6.
8. Coughlan A. K., Humphrey M. (1982), Pre-senile stroke: long term outcome for patients and their families. *Rheum. Rehab.*; **21**: 115–22.

FURTHER READING

Anonymous (1985), Management of stroke: 12 hours to 2 months, *Drug Ther. Bull.*; **23**: 9–12.

Avigad J., Jackson R., Frank A. O. (1982), Areas of social impairment in six families following stroke, *Demonstration Centres in Rehabilitation Newsletter*; **28**: 54–9.

Chamberlain M. A. (1983), Stroke rehabilitation, in *Advanced Medicine*. (Losowsky M. S., Bolton R. P., eds.) London, Royal College of Physicians of London/Pitman Books, pp. 41–7.

Field D., Cordle C. J., Bowman G. S. (1984), Coping with stroke at home, *Int. J. Rehab. Med.*; **5**: 96–100.

Humphrey M. (1985), Sexual consequences after cerebrovascular accident, *J. Roy. Soc. Med.*; **78**; 388–90.

Kendall R., Hawkins E., Meikle M. (1982), Northwick Park hospital stroke club, *Demonstration Centres in Rehabilitation Newsletter*; **28**: 78–81

Kinsella G. J., Duffy F. D. (1979), Psychosocial readjustment in the spouses of aphasic patients, *Scand. J. Rehab. Med.*; **11**: 129–32.

Legh-Smith J., Wade D. T., Langton-Hewer R. (1986), Driving after stroke, *J. Roy. Soc. Med.*; **79**; 200–3.

Robinson R. G., Price T. R. (1982). Post stroke depressive disorders: a follow up study of 103 patients, *Stroke*; **13**; 635–40.

Smith D. S., Goldenberg E., Ashburn A. et al (1981), Remedial therapy after stroke: a randomised controlled trial, *Br. Med. J.*; **282**: 517–20.

Wade D. T., Langton-Hewer R., Skilbeck C. E., David R. M. (1985), *Stroke. A Critical Approach to Diagnosis, Treatment and Management*, London, Chapman and Hall.

Wade D. T., Langton-Hewer R., Skilbeck C. E. et al. (1985), Controlled trial of a home care service for acute stroke patients. *Lancet*; **i**: 323–6.

Williams I. M. (1982), Physiotherapy 'at risk' register. *Demonstration Centres in Rehabilitation Newsletter*; **28**: 51–3.

Appendix 5.1

Keeping mobile

Mobility allowance

This is a weekly cash benefit paid to disabled people who are unable or virtually unable to walk. It is provided to enable individuals to remain mobile by paying for forms of transport more suited to their needs. It can be claimed by those between 5 and 65 years of age, and if the disability remains permanent it is continued until 75 years of age. Unfortunately a great many people are over the age of 65 when they suffer a stroke and are thus not eligible for mobility allowance (see Chapter 13).

Wheelchairs

The Department of Health and Social Security (DHSS) lends wheelchairs for indoor and outdoor use to individuals with long-term disability. These may be self-propelled or attendant-controlled, and powered or manual, although at present the DHSS does not supply outdoor self-operated powered wheelchairs. Alternatively wheelchairs can be hired or privately purchased.[1,2]

Buses

Often the height of the bus platform restricts the use of buses, though this height is lessened when the bus pulls in close to the pavement. Generally, modern buses have lower steps, hand rails and non-slip floors, and some are wheelchair-accessible.

It is best when possible to use buses out of rush hour as crowds can create difficulties for those with poor balance. Usually seats near the entrance are reserved for disabled and elderly people.

Concessionary bus fares are available to elderly and disabled people in many parts of the country, though they are often limited to travel outside peak hours.

Trains

British Rail will provide assistance for disabled individuals by meeting travellers at their departure and arrival stations and assisting them on and off the train. They prefer to have two days prior notice.

Wheelchairs can be temporarily loaned for use at the station and short-term car parking is usually available close to the station entrance.

Individuals receiving mobility allowance or attendance allowance can purchase a rail card which entitles the card holder and an accompanying adult to concessionary fares.

Taxis

Taxi cars are easier to get in and out of than London-style taxis. In London the Greater London Council introduced a scheme which has since been adopted by the majority of London boroughs whereby the holder of the taxi card is entitled to concessionary travel. A taxi card scheme also operates in other parts of the country.

Personal transport schemes

For those people who cannot manage buses and trains or ordinary access to a car, personal transport schemes enable outdoor social activities to continue. These vary considerably but almost always the cost is subsidized.

Dial-a-Ride

There are many of these schemes which involve collecting and returning individuals to their own homes using converted cars or ramped minibuses. They mainly operate in local areas but will usually include mainline railway stations.

Community Transport Scheme

These schemes are often run by voluntary organizations, again using adapted and ramped vehicles. In addition to providing voluntary drivers, some schemes lend an adapted vehicle if the disabled person can provide his or her own driver.

Returning to driving

For individuals with neurological damage affecting their perception, speed of reaction, vision and reasoning, an assessment of driving ability is necessary. There are a number of assessment centres throughout the country.[3] At Banstead Place Mobility Centre this investigation is carried out over a period of one day by a team consisting of the medical consultant, psychologist, orthotist, driving consultant, and therapist; a practical driving assessment is included and a written report is then compiled and sent to the client, general practitioner, and the hospital consultant.

Banstead Place has a demonstration area and workshop, and an authentic tarmac road system, and can allow individuals to try out various car models as well as recommending suitable adaptations.

Choosing a car

The ease with which individuals can get themselves and their wheelchairs in or out of a car can be greatly affected by door widths, seat heights, sill heights; and control layout is also important.

Car adaptations

All adaptations are VAT-exempt. A car can be adapted to be operated either entirely by hand controls, or by foot controls. For those who have difficulty in getting into a car a number of different options will help; swivel car seats, car top hoists, driving directly from the wheelchair etc. Other adaptations to make access easier include a wheelchair lift, a ramp to the rear of the vehicle and raised roof.

Motability

Motability is a scheme whereby the mobility allowance contributes towards the hiring of a new car or buying a new or used car, or wheelchair, on hire purchase. The car must be the property of, but not necessarily driven by, the disabled person.

Full details of the scheme are set out in leaflets from Motability (see Chapter 14) but the main points to note are:

1. *Hiring* – the mobility allowance is given over for 3 years in return for car rental. Extra premiums are payable according to the car model. The choice of cars is limited. The maintenance and servicing are included in the rental. A delivery charge is payable and adaptations (installation and removal) are not included.
2. *Hire purchase* – all or part of the mobility allowance is given over for the term of contract plus initial deposit, being the difference between the total mobility allowance and the total cost of the chosen vehicle. There are restrictions relating to the age and condition of a second-hand car.

Assistance and independence for the disabled (AID)

This service can be used by any disabled person even if he or she does not receive a mobility allowance to obtain a vehicle (new or second-hand) on hire purchase (see Chapter 14).

Orange badge parking scheme

This allows certain parking concessions and is available to drivers or passengers who have very considerable difficulty with mobility. Application forms and explanatory leaflets are available from the local social services department.

Vehicle excise duty exemption

This is available to those in receipt of mobility allowance or attendance allowance and who are unable or virtually unable to walk (see Chapter 13).

Rate relief

This is available for garages and car ports if the disabled owner of the vehicle is registered as physically handicapped with the local social services department.

Air and sea travel

Most airports have disabled parking spaces and wheelchairs for use within the airport and grounds. By prior arrangement, assistance can be given to both wheelchair-bound people and those with walking difficulties with boarding the plane and providing sufficient space on the plane and easy access to the toilet.

The range of facilities at UK ports varies considerably and it is advisable to check with the port manager. Assistance can be given for access to ships and with prior arrangement a lift can be used to accommodate the passenger or wheelchair.

REFERENCES

1. Department of Transport (1986). *Door to Door – A Guide to Transport for Disabled People*, 2nd ed, London, Adington.
2. Darnbrough A. Kinrade D. (1986), *Motoring and Mobility for Disabled People*, London, Royal Association of Disability and Rehabilitation (RADAR).
3. Department of Transport (1986), *Mobility, Advice and Vehicle Information Service Leaflet* (*MAVIS*), London, Department of Transport.

6

Incontinence

Christine Norton

Incontinence of urine or faeces is often the most limiting and distressing aspect of a disabling disease and may, of itself, constitute a disability for some individuals. Incontinence is a symptom rather than a diagnosis, and as such always warrants full investigation if appropriate treatment is to be possible. Sadly, at present incontinence is often accepted, by both the public and many professionals, as an inevitable accompaniment to disease or age. Many patients are simply told that it is to be expected, that they will have to learn to live with it, without investigation of the cause. Recent evidence suggests that this therapeutic pessimism is often unfounded – for the majority of people, whatever their underlying disease or disability, there can be hope of continence. At the very least most can expect some improvement in control. Even where this proves impossible, after full multidisciplinary assessment and intervention, active management should enable the individual with intractable incontinence to lead a normal life in comfort and dignity.

Continence is the ability to pass urine and faeces only in socially acceptable places. It is not an absolute – we all have to excrete body wastes, and society is geared to the excretory needs of the majority. Incontinence results when an individual does not, or cannot, comply with society's arbitrary rules. It is still commonly regarded as reflecting adversely on the moral character of the offender, causing shame, embarrassment and guilt for most sufferers. The incontinent often become socially isolated and indeed may be actively excluded from activities because of their symptoms. Where help with physical care is needed incontinence can be the deciding factor in the ability of carers to cope, or their willingness to try. Whoever the incontinent member is, the life of the whole family is disrupted. A child who wets the bed can preclude family holidays in hotels and later the adolescent may be unwilling to move away from home if the problem persists. A young mother with stress incontinence may find picking up the children, carrying heavy shopping or long journeys very difficult. An elderly incontinent relative

Table 6.1   Prevalence of urinary incontinence[1]

	15–64 years	65+ years
Men	1.6%	6.9%
Women	8.5%	11.6%

living with the family can mean that the whole house is dominated by laundry and a telltale odour, so that friends no longer visit. Thus incontinence has profound effects upon the physical, psychological and social well-being of all those who suffer from it.

Many physically disabled people find that bladder and bowel management are one of the most difficult aspects of their daily life. Often horizons are limited, not by physical abilities, but by the availability of lavatories. The uncertainty of never knowing if or when facilities will be usable, or if incontinence will occur, can make the individual unwilling to venture anywhere new, or even out of the house at all.

Incontinence is common. Because of the nature of the symptom, a majority of sufferers disguise it. Only recently has the full extent of the problem become evident. Table 6.1 shows the prevalence figures from the most comprehensive survey to date on urinary incontinence. The results were obtained from a postal survey, with the definition of 'incontinence' as leakage occurring twice or more per month.

One-fifth of those who were incontinent were judged to have a moderate to severe problem. The vast majority were not known to be incontinent by anyone in the local health or social services and even those with a severe problem were not, for the most part, receiving any help or services. Approximately one adult in 200 suffers faecal incontinence. Although incontinence is common in all age groups, the prevalence does increase with advanced old age (75 years and above), with obvious implications for an ageing population. If the majority are not now in receipt of help, the National Health Service will need to commit much greater resources in future to help those with this problem. However, it should be remembered that the majority of old people remain continent – so why should some lose this skill?

URINARY INCONTINENCE

Continence

Continence involves a complex neuromuscular co-ordination in conjunction with adequate physical and mental ability to comply with society's expectations. To be continent reliably the individual must recognize the need to micturate, appreciate the significance of that signal, be able and want to delay micturition until the correct place is reached, be able to get there and be able to void completely once there. In addition, a whole series of related skills are needed, for example locking doors, removing clothes and handwashing. Failure at any stage in this sequence can result in incontinence. For many people continence is a delicate balance. It takes only a minor alteration at any stage in the sequence to tip them either way. Assessment of an incontinent person will involve an attempt to find out where and why the balance has been disturbed. Improving continence may involve treating bladder dysfunction or increasing the individual's ability to cope with it; usually a combination of several measures will be needed, depending upon each person's unique combination of needs and problems.

Improving bladder function

Most people who wet themselves have some degree of bladder dysfunction. A careful history of urinary symptoms and a clinical examination will indicate the most likely problem. Of relevance are frequency of micturition or nocturia, urgency, stress or urge incontinence, nocturnal enuresis, dysuria and any symptoms of a voiding difficulty (such as hesitancy, straining, poor flow). Medical and drug history, and parity should be noted. Clinical examination may reveal an enlarged prostate, a loaded rectum, an atrophic vagina, pelvic floor laxity or prolapse, and any obvious neurological or other deficit. Combined with testing of the urine and measurement of the post-micturition residual urine volume, a presumptive diagnosis can usually be arrived at. Caution should be taken in ascribing diagnosis purely on the basis of current diseases – the woman with multiple sclerosis is as prone to stress incontinence as any other woman; the male stroke victim may also suffer from an enlarged prostate gland.

Where the history is not straightforward or symptoms are mixed, a variety of further laboratory or clinical investigations may be indicated. Completely accurate diagnosis of bladder dysfunction is impossible without urodynamic studies, although a working diagnosis can be made in most cases. If simple measures have failed, a mixed problem is suspected or if invasive treatment (e.g. surgery) is contemplated the patient should be referred for a cystometrogram. It is not uncommon for several separate bladder problems to co-exist, especially in those with neurological disease, and the clinician needs to be fully aware of these for treatment to be successful.

However, it is sound practice to start with the most obvious measures.

Treatment of underlying disorders (e.g. urinary tract infection, faecal impaction, diabetes or Parkinson's disease) may restore continence. Rationalization of drug therapy, especially diuretics or sedation, may reduce symptoms.

Detrusor instability

Symptoms of frequency, urgency, urge incontinence and nocturnal enuresis, in the absence of infection or post-micturition residual urine, will usually indicate detrusor instability. A cystometrogram, if performed, would show uninhibited detrusor contractions during bladder filling. Usually secondary to an upper motor neurone lesion, it may be idiopathic in the younger patient.

The most effective therapy for detrusor instability is a combination of anticholinergic medication and bladder retraining. Imipramine (e.g. 25 mg nocte or b.d.) and Oxybutinin (5 mg t.d.s.) are two of the most effective drugs amongst the many currently in use. Dry mouth and constipation can be troublesome side-effects.

Bladder retraining for urge incontinence involves the patient or carer keeping a simple record of episodes of micturition and incontinence for a baseline period of 4–7 days. The pattern is then examined and an individualized toilet pattern is worked out to anticipate incontinence and, where possible, fit in with the patient's lifestyle. Time intervals may be regular (e.g. 2-hourly) or variable (e.g. hourly in the morning after diuretics, increasing as the day progresses). The patient is asked to attempt to 'hang on' until the allotted times to pass urine. At first most find this extremely difficult and close support and encouragement are vital at this stage. As each target is achieved the time gap between toilet visits is gradually extended until, usually over a period of several weeks, a normal voiding pattern is attained – 3–4-hourly with no urgency or incontinence. The aim is both to retrain the bladder and restore the patient's confidence. Some gynaecologists will admit women to hospital for a short intensive period of retraining. Naturally the patient must be highly motivated to break the habit of frequency and to repress the urgent desire to void.

Nocturnal enuresis in children and young adults is best treated with an enuresis alarm. It is pointless just to hand out such equipment without explanation or supervision – considerable commitment is needed from child, parents and therapist for success. School nurses and health visitors often have the most experience with these alarms. Correctly used, cure rates are about 80%. The new mini alarms have made the equipment more convenient, portable and acceptable.

Stress incontinence

The symptom of leakage upon physical exertion is most commonly caused by an incompetent urethral sphincter in women. Mild stress incontinence will usually respond to pelvic floor exercises and the physiotherapist is usually the best person to teach and supervise these exercises. Women are taught to locate the pelvic floor musculature accurately (interrupting micturition mid-stream can help this) and then to contract the pelvic floor regularly (e.g. four times each hour) throughout the day. The motivated patient without gross prolapse should regain continence in 6–12 weeks. If the condition coexists with atrophic vaginitis (and hence urethritis) topical oestrogen therapy will be helpful (e.g. stilboestrol pessaries).

If prolapse or stress incontinence is severe, gynaecological help will be needed. If a woman does not wish, or is unfit, for surgery, a ring pessary may control her symptoms.

Voiding difficulties

The bladder which does not empty completely is prone to infection and the individual may experience a variety of symptoms, such as frequency (because of diminished functional capacity), difficulty in emptying and dribbling – 'overflow' incontinence. If the urethra is obstructed it may be possible to relieve this surgically, for example by prostatectomy, urethrotomy or division of a stricture. A long-standing obstruction can lead to a superimposed detrusor hypertrophy and instability, and so masquerade as urge incontinence. Severe faecal impaction will often cause a mechanical obstruction.

Alternatively, the problem may be an atonic bladder which does not contract effectively (e.g. in diabetes) or detrusor–sphincter dyssynergia, in which co-ordination of the voiding sequence is lost (common in many neurological diseases). The treatment of choice is intermittent clean self-catheterization (ICSC). This technique is widely used with patients with a spinal injury or spina bifida, many of whom are now avoiding a urinary diversion. It is now gaining recognition in many other fields. The patient is taught, using a clean (not aseptic) technique, to introduce a simple plastic catheter into the bladder in order to drain out the residuum which cannot be voided. For very young children the parents are taught at first, but from the age of 8 years onwards most people can learn ICSC. Where physical or mental impairment preclude this, a carer may learn. After each use the catheter is washed and re-used for about 1 week. Because the bladder is being emptied completely and many of the domestic micro-organisms encountered are relatively benign, significant infection is rare. Some patients void exclusively by intermittent catheter and so introduce it 4–6 times per day, or even less, to drain off a gradually accumulating residuum. This management is also proving effective for some demented patients who have unco-ordinated voiding, where a carer is available and willing to catheterize.

If ICSC is impossible (e.g. in a quadriplegic) often the only way to protect renal function is to destroy continence completely by surgically dividing the urethral sphincter.

IMPROVING THE ABILITY TO COPE WITH BLADDER FUNCTION

Many simple measures can be tried to improve the patient's ability to cope with either normal or abnormal bladder function.

Mobility

Anything which improves mobility will enable the patient to reach the lavatory more quickly and reliably. This is especially important for those with urgency. This might include treating a disease impeding mobility (e.g. Parkinson's disease); making walking less painful (e.g. prescribing analgesia for arthritis); provision of a suitable walking aid; or attention to the feet or footwear (pp. 25–9). Referral to the physiotherapist or chiropodist might be relevant. Good eyesight is also vital for mobility, and sometimes measures to improve continence can be as seemingly remote as obtaining a new pair of spectacles! The occupational therapist can advise on suitable furniture if rising from a bed or chair is difficult, and may teach the patient or relatives techniques for safe and effective transfer.

Room layout can be significant in helping or hindering mobility. A cluttered room with loose mats and narrow doorways will impede access to the lavatory. A walking aid may be inappropriate or counterproductive if it cannot be manoeuvred in the space available.

Dexterity

Poor manual dexterity may mean that reaching the lavatory is not sufficient to ensure continence. Considerable agility of the hands is needed to remove clothing, position, cleanse and correctly replace clothes. Trousers with button-up openings, multiple layers of clothing and complicated incontinence appliances can add to the problem. Judicious use of velcro fastenings, wrap-over shirts and split-crotch pants can make access easier and quicker. Toilet rolls are particularly difficult for the hemiplegic patient and pull-out boxes of toilet tissue, if positioned with forethought, are much easier. A bottom wiper can prevent soiling for those with limited arm movements.

The lavatory

In the home it may be possible to design the lavatory to suit the needs of a disabled person and many different layouts are available for different needs. A variety of grab-rails, surrounds, raised seats and other modifications are possible. Good lighting will help the partially sighted. Warmth and a comfortable seat may encourage more complete voiding. An outward-opening door can increase space for a wheelchair or walking frame and consideration should be given to whether approach is easiest laterally, forwards, or at an angle. If the patient can no longer get to an existing lavatory a grant may be obtained for the cost of a purpose-built one (e.g. downstairs), where this fits in with the other domestic arrangements. Social services are responsible for the provision of aids to daily living and independence and a social worker can advise on obtaining the available assistance.

Lavatory access may be much more of a problem to the disabled person outside the home. Despite public policy and some improvements, provision is inadequate in many public and employment situations. Both continent and incontinent disabled people find this limits their activities.

Alternatives to the lavatory

If the lavatory cannot be reached then a substitute may be used, at home or when out. The most familiar is the male urinal, or 'bottle'. Available in lightweight plastic with a snap-on lid or non-spill adaptor, this can be used by most men in lying, sitting or standing positions. A completely disposable non-spill urinal is particularly useful on long journeys for men with frequency. Extending the opening of trousers down to the crotch seam makes a bottle much easier to use. Various hand-held female urinals are also available and can be used in bed, or seated, by the reasonably dextrous woman. A standard bedpan is probably the most difficult to use. Many individual remedies have been found – a narrow fridge jug is useful for women with limited hip abduction and can be used standing by women who find sitting difficult or painful. For the wheelchair-bound person who cannot transfer, a foam cushion with a cut-out slit and a receptacle underneath to collect urine (or faeces) is discreet and can avoid hours of sitting on wet clothes or pads.

Most health authorities will provide a commode for people with limited mobility (although some leave this to voluntary bodies such as the Red Cross, or have a long waiting list). It can never be presumed that a commode will be acceptable, in living or sleeping areas. Many people are embarrassed to use a commode in the bedroom, if shared with a spouse, and prefer to struggle to the lavatory, even if this is downstairs or outside. A commode requires emptying, and responsibility for this should be clarified prior to delivery if the patient cannot manage. Some commodes can be disguised as an ordinary chair; others have wheels for easy movement. Removable side-arms may help transfer from a wheelchair. Some convert into a Sani-chair which can be wheeled over the lavatory; others can be clamped to the side of the bed for safer transfer. Even selection of a commode must take individual needs into account. If emptying is a problem, a portable chemical toilet may be more suitable.

Toilet programmes

Some people visit the lavatory remarkably infrequently and only ever go at the last possible moment. If such a person is also immobile, has an unstable bladder or is forgetful then simple teaching, combined with keeping a chart, and the use of clocks or timers, may enable a toilet pattern to be established which anticipates impending micturition. Those with impaired bladder sensation should develop a habit of voiding by the clock. Many people do not realize that warning time is considerably reduced with advancing age, or that nocturia becomes the norm and must be allowed for.

Patients with advanced dementia may exhibit no discernible pattern to their incontinence and if this is so it is best to advise carers to take the individual to the toilet at pre-set intervals on a regular basis in an attempt to prevent as much incontinence as possible.

The mentally impaired

The mentally impaired – whether confused, mentally handicapped, or demented – may be incontinent because of lack of social awareness, or because mental capacity cannot cope with the complex sequence of skills necessary for continence, or because of a bladder dysfunction. A psychologist, community psychiatric nurse or the mental handicap team may often help in assessment and planning of care.

A great deal of success can be achieved using behaviour modification techniques with mentally handicapped people of any age. Toilet training is particularly successful if started early and if family or carers are enthusiastic. Indeed, in some cases this will enable community care for someone who could not be managed at home if incontinent. By devising an individualized programme which rewards the desired behaviour (continence) and gradually suppresses the incontinence, most even profoundly mentally handicapped people can eventually achieve continence.

The demented patient may respond to simple, repetitive teaching and reality orientation. Often the family can be taught how to maximize the patient's remaining level of functioning. It is important not just to accept incontinence as inevitable in dementia, as it is usually one of the last social skills to be lost and is often caused by reversible problems (e.g. faecal impaction, infection, detrusor instability). Even in advanced dementia relatives may be alerted to the non-verbal signals of impending micturition exhibited by many people, for example agitation, and so be able to maintain continence in someone they know well.

Incontinence may also be a feature of psychiatric disturbance, notably depression. It is difficult to disentangle cause and effect in the cycle of depression, apathy, isolation and incontinence. Once established, the patient has little motivation to attempt continence. In some instances those trying to help may unwittingly reinforce the cycle by 'rewarding' incontinence with attention, which was not forthcoming when the individual was continent. Improving the social environment may increase motivation (e.g. attendance at a day centre or some other activity). The incontinence and depression may need separate treatment.

MANAGEMENT OF INTRACTABLE INCONTINENCE

Despite the very best in available treatment a minority of patients will remain incontinent to some degree. For these people good management is the key to enabling a relatively normal lifestyle with the minimum of discomfort or embarrassment.

One of the most important elements of care is support and counselling for the individual and his or her family. It is vital for the incontinent person to feel accepted and opportunity must be given for frank discussion of problems. It is often difficult for people to express their feelings and fears about such an intimate subject – indeed some lack vocabulary even to start talking – and considerable trust and rapport must be built up if the health professional is to offer optimal support. It is unhelpful to dismiss worries with reassuring platitudes: 'Of course you don't smell' convinces no one. Teaching the patient about normal and abnormal bladder and bowel physiology and giving an explanation of why incontinence occurs often aids understanding and facilitates management. Ignorance and misconceptions are common and can lead to extraordinary, often counterproductive practices. If the patient and family understand the condition they are much more able to participate actively and contribute to management.

Often very simple and seemingly obvious advice is the most effective. A reasonable (e.g. 1½ litre) fluid intake in 24 hours should be encouraged, but the timing of this can be adjusted to anticipate problems, e.g. restricting fluids before an outing. Timing of medication, especially diuretics, is important, and sometimes a divided dose is more easily coped with. General health advice on diet, avoiding constipation and keeping mobile will help.

If the patient is dependent, support for relatives can make the difference between community and residential care. The difficulties and unpleasantness of caring for a heavily incontinent person in the home should never be underestimated. Relatives are often left feeling both guilty and inadequate and reassurance that they are doing the best possible, together with relevant practical support, and if applicable regular holiday relief (see pp. 188, 256), will enable them to cope better and for longer.

INCONTINENCE AIDS

There are a bewildering variety of incontinence aids available. No one aid is suitable for the needs of all incontinent people and choice should be tailored to suit each individual's abilities and incontinence. Factors such as volume, timing and type of incontinence, self-help skills, activities, anatomy, personal preference and cost must all be considered when selecting an aid. Many companies are only just realizing the huge potential market for incontinence aids and the next few years will see a great expansion in the quality and quantity of items available.

Pads and pants

The majority of incontinent people use absorbent padding worn inside retaining pants. In the UK, pads and pants are not available on prescription and are usually supplied free of charge via the district nursing services. Unfortunately, supply varies greatly between districts and which items are likely to be available very much depends on where the patient lives. Some districts provide a good range, with facilities to make special orders for exceptional needs and a regular, efficient delivery service. Others provide only one or two low-cost (and often low-quality) items, ration supplies regardless of individual needs and have no delivery service, so that those who cannot collect have difficulties obtaining anything.

In practice, many incontinent people buy their own pads, either because they do not seek help, or none is forthcoming. Sanitary towels are the most easily available, but while they are small and discreet, they will only cope with minimal leakage and can prove very expensive for those on a limited income.

Plastic pants were once the only available protective garment. Their use should be avoided as they cause so many skin problems, as well as being hot, noisy, uncomfortable and undignified. They have been superseded by both the Kanga-style pants, which have a one-way fabric with a waterproof pouch to hold the pad, and by the great range of plastic-backed pads, which are usually held in place by stretch mesh pants. The better pads are made from high-quality pulp, which is very absorbent and does not crumble in use. Many manufacturers are aware of patient preferences and are attempting to make the products more aesthetically pleasing and acceptable to users; for instance, by designing pants to look like normal underwear and using plain wrappers. For the very heavily incontinent, all-in-one diaper systems (large versions of babies' disposable nappies), although infantilizing, are often the best option. Pads are available in a variety of sizes, shapes, thicknesses and absorbences and one can be found to suit most needs.

Bed protection

The patient with nocturnal enuresis needs some way of protecting the bed and linen from soiling. A fitted plastic mattress cover will save the mattress, but can be hot to sleep on. A variety of waterproof, disposable or washable, drawsheets are available. The cheap 5-ply bed pad in common use does little to protect the patient or bed from any but minimal leakage. Some body-worn pads are now being developed specifically for night use and are often more comfortable and functional.

Appliances

Various collection devices can be used for the male who is incontinent of urine. None are suitable for the female. Dribble pouches are simple, disposable or re-usable, and fit over the penis to cope with small amounts of leakage. Penile sheaths are the most suitable device for many incontinent men, provided that they are reasonably dextrous and do not have a retracted penis. A sheath is best secured in place by an adhesive strip, or medical adhesive to attach it directly to the penis, and then is connected to a leg bag to collect the urine. For the man who cannot manage a sheath or has a retracted penis, a pubic pressure or other body-worn urinal may be used. As these are both complicated and expensive they should be fitted by an appliance expert in the first instance. Most of the male appliances are available on prescription.

SKIN CARE

Advice on skin care is important to help the individual to be comfortable and free from pressure sores. Remarkably, the majority of incontinent people have few skin problems, providing they are in good general health and maintain good personal hygiene. It is best simply to wash the skin with soap and water and dry it thoroughly with a soft towel. Heavily scented soaps and talcum powder should be avoided, as should making the skin soggy by the over-use of creams. Many rashes are the result of a skin sensitivity to preparations used rather than contact with urine. If the skin does become sore, the cause should be discovered – an appliance may be too tight, a pad may be irritating or there may be an infection present. Small amounts of a suitable cream. (e.g. Sudocrem) can be used if the skin is actually sore.

If washing and personal hygiene are a problem the district nurse or bath attendant may be able to offer help.

ODOUR

The most common worry of incontinent people is that they smell offensive. In our odour-conscious society any hint of bodily functions is taboo. In practice, freshly voided urine should smell little and few incontinent people have a problem, so long as hygiene is adequate. If urine is offensive it is probably infected or over-concentrated. An effective aid should contain urine and prevent contamination of clothes, furniture and floors. Clothes should be chosen in easily laundered fabrics. Soiled pads or laundry should be kept in closed containers (e.g. a plastic bin with a fitting lid) until they can be dealt with. Ventilation will help to disperse any odours. If the patient does have an odour problem several specifically designed deodorants are available on prescription.

RELATIONSHIPS

Interpersonal relations often become strained if one partner is incontinent. The patient may feel sexually unattractive, and generally that he or she is a burden to the partner. Many incontinent women find that they leak during sexual intercourse or at orgasm and this can be very inhibiting. Recognition that this may be an area of tension and enabling open discussion of problems may help a couple to reach some solutions.

CATHETERIZATION

The use of an indwelling urethral catheter to manage intractable incontinence has to some extent been discredited. However, while a catheter should always be seen very much as a last resort and only considered where all else has failed to cure or cope with the incontinence, there can be no doubt that selected patients can benefit enormously. If incontinence is severe enough to restrict activities, the patient can experience a greatly enhanced quality of life with a catheter. Each decision has to be made for each individual's circumstances.

The major drawback to long-term catheterization is inevitable infection. There is no way of preventing chronic infection from a shifting spectrum of micro-organisms. For this reason the younger patient with a good life expectancy should only be catheterized for exceptional reasons. Alternatives such as intermittent self-catheterization or, more rarely, a urinary diversion are often preferable. Infection can only be eradicated for short periods and so to avoid emergence of multiresistant organisms the best policy is only to treat symptomatic infection, i.e. if the patient becomes pyrexial, unwell, has loin pain or is unexplainedly confused.

The success of catheter management depends to some extent on the correct choice of catheter. A small size (14 or 16 French gauge) with a small balloon (5–10 ml) made from silicone or silicone-coated latex is associated with fewer problems. The shorter female-length catheter may be more manageable and discreet for ladies. Larger catheters are only needed if the urine is full of debris, and generally cause problems of discomfort and stricture and may aggravate an unstable bladder, with consequent bladder spasms and leakage. If a catheter leaks frequently, anticholinergic medications may dampen down detrusor contractions and bypassing. A smaller catheter or a smaller balloon may also help.

Some patients repeatedly block a catheter. A good fluid intake (2–3 litres in 24 hours), mobility and avoiding constipation may help. If not, regular washouts may be tried. A washout regimen should be devised to suit the individual. Most patients find that 2–3 washouts with normal saline or sterile water (100–200 ml) per week suffice, but this can be done daily if necessary. Proprietary preparations for washouts offer little advantage over water, and repeated use of antimicrobial solutions may encourage the emergence of resistant strains of organisms. If blocking persists the catheter will have to be changed more often than the 2–3 months possible for most patients.

It is important to remember that the patient has to live with a catheter 24 hours a day. Good teaching can enable the individual to be confident in handling it. The collection bag must be convenient and easy to disguise under clothing, e.g. in a leg bag or a bag attached to a waist belt or worn in a pocket in specially designed pants, trousers or skirt. It is usual to change this for a larger bag at night so that sleep is not disturbed.

If the patient is sexually active advice should be given on how to cope with the catheter. Women can usually maintain an active sex life with a catheter in situ. Some find that a change of position during intercourse increases comfort. It is best to advise men with a urethral catheter to avoid intercourse, although a few do continue sexual activity. It is sometimes feasible to teach the patient or partner to remove and replace the catheter. A suprapubic catheter might be a better alternative and should be considered for the long-term management of sexually active men who need catherization.

SERVICES AND BENEFITS

The incontinent person may be able to make use of a variety of services and benefits. Attendance allowance may be payable if a carer is needed to help with toilet duties or incontinence. A home help can help, especially with laundry. Some districts have an 'incontinence laundry service' which collects from the home. Sometimes a grant can be obtained for exceptional need, e.g. to install a washing machine or to replace ruined furniture. Some authorities have a pad delivery service and/or collection service. A social worker can advise the patient on his or her entitlements and how to go about claiming them.

FAECAL INCONTINENCE

Faecal incontinence, although much less common than urinary incontinence, can be even more devastating when it does occur. There are many possible physiological causes, such as severe diarrhoea, neurogenic bowel, muscle impairment and bowel disease, as well as environmental and psychological factors similar to those for urinary incontinence. Any change in bowel habit warrants full investigation as it may herald serious underlying pathology. However, the commonest cause of faecal incontinence is severe constipation with impaction of faeces, and overflow incontinence which may be of formed stool or spurious diarrhoea from mucus seepage. If the rectum is permanently loaded the anal sphincter will become patulous and allow free passage of faecal matter. Faeces are palpable in the rectum in the majority of cases. A course of enemas, often 7–10, is needed to disimpact the bowel and for many this will resolve the incontinence and measures must then be introduced to prevent recurrence.

Patients with neurological disease may be faecally incontinent because of a failure to inhibit reflex contractions of the colon and rectum (similar to detrusor instability in the bladder). Such patients may, if sensible or carefully supervised, be managed by artificially inducing constipation with a constipating agent and then planning evacuation using suppositories or an enema at convenient intervals (see p. 175).

Surgical repair may be indicated for patients who have lost the anorectal angle. For patients with severe uncontrollable faecal incontinence a colostomy (see Chapter 11) may make a significant improvement to their quality of life.

THE URODYNAMIC CLINIC AND CONTINENCE ADVISER

Some districts are now developing specialist services for the investigation and treatment of incontinence. We believe that all incontinent people should have access to such facilities when needed. Urodynamic studies are an invaluable aid to diagnosis where this is in doubt. However, as incontinence is such a common problem, it will remain unrealistic to expect such clinics to see every incontinent patient. This is neither necessary nor desirable. Many incontinence problems can be resolved by effective co-operation of the multidisciplinary primary care team. The post of continence nurse adviser has evolved in some places to act as a clinical support and resource person to the team.

REFERENCES

1. Thomas T. et al (1980), Prevalence of urinary incontinence, *Br. Med. J.*; 28: 1243–5.

FURTHER READING

Association of Continence Advisers (1988), *Directory of Continence and Toiletting Aids*, 2nd ed, London, ACA.

Avery Jones F., Godding E. W. (1972), *Management of Constipation*, Oxford, Blackwell Scientific Publications.

Disabled Living Foundation, *Notes on Incontinence*, London, DLF.

Drug Tarrif Supplement (1983), *Advisory List of Urinary Incontinence Appliances*, London, DHSS.

Mandelstam D. (1986), *Incontinence and its Management*, 2nd ed. London, Croom Helm.

Meadow R. (1983), *Help for Bedwetting*, Edinburgh, Churchill Livingstone.

Morgan R. (1980), *Childhood Incontinence*, London, Disabled Living Foundation.

Norton C. S. (1986), *Nursing for continence*, Beaconsfield Publishers, Beaconsfield.

Smith P., Smith L. (1987), *Continence and Incontinence Psychological Approaches to Development and Treatment*. London, Croom Helm.

Stanton S. L. (1977), *Female Urinary Incontinence*, London, Lloyd-Luke.

Willington F. L. (1976), *Incontinence in the Elderly*, London, Academic Press.

7

Multiple disabilities

Malcolm Hodkinson

Though multiple disabilities may occur in patients of any age, multiple pathology is particularly common in the elderly. The management of multiple disabilities will therefore be considered in the specific context of the older patient, although the principles illustrated can equally well apply to younger patients.

What patterns of multiple disability are encountered? Patterns of disability can be described only in a very general way for it is true to say that there are as many patterns as there are patients! However, we can usefully consider disabilities under a number of broad headings: physical, mental and social.

PHYSICAL DISABILITIES

Firstly, physical disabilities may be the consequence of acute disease processes and thus have a good chance of being short-lived and reversible. For example, left- or right-sided heart failure, chest infections, urinary tract infections and other such common acute diseases in the elderly patient may powerfully contribute to current disability because of consequent malaise, fatigue, weakness or dyspnoea as a result of the impact of the disease on exercise tolerance. These potentially temporary disabilities are likely to have powerful interactions with pre-existing disabilities to which the patient may hitherto have been well compensated. In this situation, a previously relatively active old person may become totally compromised so that early and effective rehabilitation must be coupled with the medical treatment of his or her acute disease process. Probably the most important consequence of the development of the specialty of geriatric medicine has been to make this essential aspect of the management of elderly patients more widely appreciated. Equally, this need to unite immediate rehabilitation with the treatment of acute disease underlies the necessity for an effective geriatric service to be based in the district general hospital, not only so that elderly patients are appropriately managed from the very beginning of their stay, but also so that through example and effective liaison these principles are applied wherever patients with multiple disabilities are admitted within the hospital.

Secondly, a new and perhaps major disability may occur acutely, for example a cerebrovascular accident or a fracture. Here similar principles apply; rehabilitation needs to start straight away and the rehabilitation plans must take full account of the pre-existing disabilities. We may also have to deal with major psychological consequences of the sudden onset of major disability such as anxiety, anger or depression.

Chronic physical disorders may contribute to disability in a similar way to acute intercurrent illness. So, for example, chronic cardiac failure or chronic obstructive airways disease may seriously impair exercise tolerance whilst a host of other conditions may have a major impact because of their constitutional effects and consequent malaise, debility, fatigue and weakness. Alternatively, chronic conditions may have a more specific effect, as is particularly the case with many conditions of the nervous system or locomotor system. Here common examples are osteoarthritis, a virtually ubiquitous condition in the elderly; rheumatoid arthritis which is usually 'burnt out' in the older age group, parkinsonism and the residual disabilities from old fractures and cerebrovascular accidents. There may be unfortunate pairing of disabilities, for example osteoarthritis of the knees is likely to be far more disabling when coupled with obesity in an elderly woman – an all too common situation.

Sensory problems are very common in old age and poor vision and hearing are given great weight by the elderly when assessing their own overall disability. Regrettably, health professionals are likely to pay far less attention to these problems than is warranted. Deafness is an important barrier to rehabilitation by virtue of the problems of communication which arise between patient and therapist. Provision of hearing aids can be of great benefit but the full potential will only be achieved if there is proper instruction, encouragement and follow-up. Visual problems may be remediable if due to cataract or not if due to retinal degenerative conditions. Severely impaired vision has an obvious impact on overall activities of daily living performance but in addition poor vision and hearing independently, or more potently when combined, make the development of mental confusion far more likely.[1]

Speech problems may also present considerable obstacles to rehabilitation as well being major disabilities in their own right. Dysphasia is particularly important and may not only compromise the patient's ability to cope in his or her own home but also greatly reduces the prospects of successful integration into old people's homes or other institutional forms of care.

MENTAL DISABILITIES

Mental disabilities are extremely common in elderly patients, particularly among those admitted to hospital.[1] Perhaps commonest of all are the confusional states, associated with so many acute medical illnesses but most strikingly with infections, especially of the respiratory or urinary tracts, with left heart failure or with carcinomatosis. The adverse effects of drugs, particularly those with central nervous system actions such as sedatives, tranquillizers, antidepressants and antiparkinsonian agents, also give rise to confusional states. Whilst these side-effects are typically of short duration, this depends entirely on the reversibility of the underlying physical precipitant and if this condition is persistent the confusional state may be subacute or chronic and closely mimic dementia. Dementia is also quite common and those with dementia seem to be particularly vulnerable to the development of superadded confusional states, whether from acute intercurrent illness or from injudicious use of drugs. Dementia is most often of the Alzheimer type, although multi-infarct dementia (arteriosclerotic dementia) is also quite common, as is a mixture of the two.

Confusion is thus commonplace, whether from dementia, confusional state or a combination of the two. It has an obvious and major contribution to overall disability and perhaps an even greater impact on the capacity for successful response to rehabilitation. Simple assessment scales which test orientation and memory are widely used in geriatric practice[2,3] and are of great practical value both in the initial assessment of the patient and in monitoring subsequent progress.

Confusion may also have considerable implications with regard to carers. Sanford[4] has shown that carers found behavioural disturbance such as wandering and noisiness particularly hard to bear and that incontinence, particularly incontinence of faeces (pp. 156–7), was also a major reason for home care being abandoned.

Depression is also a frequent finding among elderly patients and must not be overlooked in view of the prospects for successful treatment. Unrelieved, depression may prove a powerful barrier to rehabilitation.

Other psychiatric conditions such as paraphrenia are far less common. However, the personality of the patient is always an important consideration. Motivation is perhaps the most powerful influence on the success of rehabilitation and a personality lacking drive and motivation can be considered to be a most important disability with a major impact on the overall performance of that patient.

Personality may also be important in other ways. Some elderly patients are grossly unrealistic with regard to plans for their future and this may greatly complicate their management. They may be unwilling to accept necessary help and fail to recognize their disability and vulnerability. Others may be over-dependent and expect an unreasonable amount of help, totally failing to recognize the strains this imposes on friends and neighbours. Often this is coupled with highly manipulative behaviour which may rapidly alienate helpers. Other personalities again may gain far more help than they need by being so amiable and grateful that willing helpers find themselves doing more and more until a point is reached when they can no longer cope with a totally unnecessary burden.

Alcoholism is a fairly frequent problem in the elderly, particularly those living in isolation, and not only creates medical problems in its own right but may also serve to alienate caring friends or relatives.

Occasionally, intellectually well preserved old people may deliberately withdraw from all social contacts and allow themselves to retreat into conditions of considerable squalor – the so-called senile squalor syndrome or Diogenes syndrome – and it can be extremely difficult to intervene successfully in such a situation.

SOCIAL DISABILITIES

Social disabilities of elderly patients may be many. The elderly often occupy unsatisfactory accommodation. Because of their inability to afford more expensive housing, they may live in inconvenient, old and poorly maintained flats or houses which may be damp, poorly heated or with inadequate sanitary or other amenities. Alternatively, an old person or elderly couple may continue to live in their old family house which is now far too large for them and which they cannot therefore maintain adequately. There may be specific problems such as steps and stairs, uneven floors or unsafe floor coverings and old and perhaps dangerous electrical wiring or appliances. Rehousing may solve these problems but, unless the new house is very close to the old accommodation, serious new problems may be created by severing supportive links with neighbours which have been built up over many years. Rehousing in so-called sheltered accommodation, in a specially designed small flat in a group of such units with a resident warden to check that all is well each day, may help fill the gap resulting from loss of former neighbourhood support.

Neighbours are particularly important for many old people, especially the very elderly, who may have no close relatives or friends to care for them. Those relatives who do exist may live too far away or may themselves be old and disabled. Elderly women who have outlived their husbands or who never married are particularly disadvantaged and are grossly over-represented among those who are in permanent institutional care.

It is very important that management plans for old people with multiple disability should take full regard of the importance of the supporting social network and not overlook the strength of the informal help available from neighbours, friends and acquaintances. It may often be preferable to make the best of what may be basically inadequate accommodation and preserve social links rather than press for rehousing. Such adaptations can be instituted by the local authority far more rapidly than rehousing can be accomplished. Local authorities employ domiciliary occupational therapists to advise on the most suitable adaptations that will enable the disabled person to continue to manage in his or her own home (see pp. 20–4, 123–5).

It must be recognized that even a strong supporting network may weaken or disappear when the old person is absent for any length of time so that in-patient rehabilitation is always a race against time; if the rehabilitation takes too long the increased social dehiscence will more than outweigh the extra gains in activities of daily living. Therapeutic greed can thus have disastrous effects and the alternative to early discharge may well be no discharge at all.

OLD AGE

Perhaps old age in its own right should not be accepted as a disability. However, there are many age-associated minor changes which may not warrant a separate diagnosis but nonetheless make important contributions to overall disability. Thus on the physical level might be listed the poorer strength, endurance, speed and agility that are commonplace in old age. Balance and co-ordination are less efficient. Mentally, though intellectually well preserved, old people may have a more rigid approach in adapting to disability and are slower to learn new ways, at least if these are taught in a way which is better suited to younger people. The disengagement which is such a common feature of the mental approach to life of the very elderly may make it more difficult for them to battle against a new disability and they may react with resigned acceptance which precludes effective rehabilitation.

MULTIFACTORIAL NATURE OF DISABILITY

We have examined the likelihood of multiple pathology in the elderly person. These multiple disorders may often present as a single clinical problem which is essentially of multifactorial aetiology. Such rather non-specific presentations as falls, failing social competence, deteriorating mobility, confusion or incontinence are thus commonplace. It is vital that these are not simply put down to old age. Effective management must be based on adequate diagnosis embracing physical, mental and social dimensions. However, the mere elaboration of a long string of diagnoses is not what is needed. Health workers must identify the key issues so that treatment may be concentrated appropriately and a realistic prognosis may be made based on effective plans for the patient's future made in consultation with the patient, family or other carers.

The need for a multidisciplinary approach

Multiple pathology and multifactorial disability make it essential to combine the skills of all relevant caring professions. This multidisciplinary approach is vital both for effective diagnosis and assessment and for the formulation of sound management plans in consultation with the patient. The case conference technique, where all relevant professionals – doctors, nurses, occupational therapists, physiotherapists, speech therapists and social workers particularly – can pool their information and expertise and jointly formulate management plans, is now an integral part of clinical practice in departments of geriatric medicine and many other units dealing with patients with multiple disabilities. Regular and effective case conferences are one important aspect of a successful rehabilitation team but close co-operation and good communication between team members need to be maintained continuously. There must be especially good communication with the patient and, after he or she leaves hospital, there must be good feedback on subsequent progress. This self-monitoring is needed both to correct any organizational problems in the delivery of aftercare which may occur and also so that the team can learn and build up its expertise.

It is equally important that the rehabilitation team should not be too hospital-oriented but rather should build the strongest possible community links. It must ensure that information available in the community from the general practitioner, the home help service or community nursing service, for example, is fully collated and used. It is often of considerable help, particularly when a patient has been in hospital for a longer than average time or has severe disabilities, to make appropriate home visits in order to assess accurately the practical problems which will affect the patient's daily living and what might be done to improve matters. Most often such visits will be carried out by occupational therapists together with the patient, though other members of the team may sometimes more appropriately be involved (see pp. 123–5).

COMMUNITY SUPPORT

The facilities available in the community are more fully described on pp. 191–3 and in Chapter 13. In view of this, the present account will concentrate on the relevance of these services to the care of disabled elderly people without going into details of their nature and organization.

The development of a complex network of supporting services in the community has been an important aspect of health and social services in Britain and has underpinned the development of modern geriatric medicine and allowed the large majority of disabled elderly people to return home after hospital admission. There has been a fear that such extensive provision of formal services would encourage relatives to do less for the elderly, thus undermining the informal caring networks which depend on these relatives, neighbours and friends. International comparisons do not support this view. It seems more probable that relatives and other carers are supported and not supplanted by the adequate provision of these services. Certainly good management plans should attempt to integrate the statutory and informal supports together into an effective whole. Three services are of particular importance and will be considered further here – home helps, meals on wheels and community nursing.

Home helps

Home helps have the elderly as their largest client group. Typically, home helps are mature women with a considerable fund of life experience who are unburdened by any unnecessary over-professionalization. Their main function is to undertake those domestic tasks which their client cannot manage, such as general housework, cooking, shopping and laundry. However, a special strength of the support they give is that they often do so much more than this. They often develop very close emotional ties with their client, becoming a key figure in their life and an effective surrogate daughter both in practical and emotional terms. They thus provide the cornerstone of the support system which enables so many old and disabled people to manage successfully in their own homes (see also pp. 255–6).

Meals on wheels

This too can be a valuable service, providing a daily hot meal to those unable to cook adequately themselves. However, though there is the human contact with the person delivering the meal, this is necessarily brief so that close relationships and therefore useful emotional support are far less likely to develop than is the case with home helps. This 'hit and run' aspect of the meals on wheels service limits its value considerably (see pp. 255–6).

Community nursing

Community nurses again have the elderly as their largest client group. They are a very important part of the support system and may undertake a wide range of nursing duties (pp. 191–3). The most common tasks include bathing, helping very disabled patients in and out of bed and technical procedures such as dressings, bowel care, giving injections or supervising medication. They have an important role in the management of incontinence, providing aids such as marsupial pants, incontinence pads and devices, or performing catheterization when required. Increasingly, community nurses are attached to a specific general practice and become an important part of the primary health care team, able to give effective feedback to the general practitioner if there are significant changes in the patient's condition.

In addition to these and other similar services operating in the elderly person's own home, there are a wealth of other facilities in the community. Thus luncheon clubs, provided an elderly person is capable of attending them, have a definite advantage over meals on wheels as they have a far greater social benefit, allowing the old person to get out and about and meet other people in a friendly atmosphere as well as providing a cheap and nutritious meal. Local authority day centres may also provide a major social stimulus to lonely and disabled old people. Attendance may also afford much needed relief to a carer who has a free day to do shopping or pursue his or her own social life, which may otherwise be severely restricted.

In organizing social support for disabled old people we must aim to provide the right amount of help. Too much may be worse than too little, since over-provision of help encourages dependence and can rapidly destroy all that has been, perhaps laboriously, achieved by rehabilitation. Skills need to be practised if they are to be maintained so meals on wheels should not be provided for people who are capable of cooking for themselves, for example. If there is doubt as to whether some form of help is needed, the situation should be monitored closely rather than providing the service 'just to be sure'.

AFTERCARE

When an old person with multiple disabilities is discharged from hospital after a period of inpatient treatment, it is not enough merely to organize a sizeable package of social service support; effective medical follow-up must also be ensured. This is of particular importance in the period immediately following discharge when people are still in the process of re-establishing themselves at home and they are at their most vulnerable.

It is also a time of handover of clinical responsibility from hospital consultant to the patient's own general practitioner. It is therefore of the utmost importance that there should be effective communication from hospital to general practitioner. Letters must be prompt and give sufficient detail, including the level of independence achieved by the patient and the social support which has been arranged for him or her. Where discharge arrangements are more complicated, they need to be made in consultation with the general practitioner and a telephone communication prior to discharge will be needed. Formal follow-up may be arranged from the hospital in the form of outpatient or day hospital attendance or visits to the patient at home by health visitor or specialist geriatric nurse visitor. Such arrangements can be of great value but it is vital that they are organized so that they do not confuse clinical responsibility. The general practitioner and primary health care team are now clinically responsible for the patient and this needs to be clear to all concerned. Specialist follow-up and advice from the hospital must support the general practitioner in the care of the patient at home and must not unwittingly usurp his clinical responsibility. Follow-up which is based on the primary health care team, perhaps by community nurse or attached health visitor, may be more appropriate as it will avoid this pitfall.

REFERENCES

1. Hodkinson H. M. (1973), Mental impairment in the elderly, *J. Roy. Coll. Phys. (Lon.)*; 7: 305–17.
2. Denham M. J., Jeffreys P. M. (1972), Routine mental assessment in elderly patients, *Mod. Geriatr.*; 2: 275–9.
3. Hodkinson H. M. (1972). Evaluation of a mental test score for assessment of mental impairment in the elderly, *Age Ageing*; 1: 233–8.
4. Sanford J. R. A. (1975), Tolerance of disability in elderly dependants by supporters at home: its significance for hospital patients, *Br. Med. J.*; 3: 471.

8

Multiple sclerosis

Sandy Burnfield and Andrew Frank

Multiple sclerosis (MS) is a devastating disease for patients, their families and friends, and also for the caring professions who try and help those suffering from its effects. Prevalence varies between areas, but in the UK is more than 60 per 100 000 population. There will be approximately 100–200 patients in the average health district, and a general practitioner can expect to have at least 1–2 patients in his or her care.

Living with MS is complicated by a number of factors: the difficulty in establishing the diagnosis with certainty; the uncertainty of the prognosis for the individual patient, at least in the early stages; the problem of relapse and remission which is a characteristic of this condition for many patients (Fig. 8.1); the lack of any effective curative treatment (despite many unjustified claims); and the diversity of symptoms and disabilities resulting from multiple plaques of demyelination.

These factors complicate management for the caring professions. Many general practitioners have little experience of the disease, and neurologists, swamped by the busy clinics, are unable to focus time on patients for whom no treatment is proven to alter the established course of the disease.

Since doctors have been trained to function with a 'disease intervention' pattern of management, many feel ill-equipped to help those with a disease whose course they cannot effectively alter. Much can be done, however, to help those suffering from this disease to lead a fuller life than might have been expected.

Only a small proportion of people with MS proceed eventually to severe disability. There is little information which might help answer the questions asked by newly diagnosed individuals on how disabled they will be in 5, 10 or 20 years' time. Many patients remain independent 20 years after the diagnosis is made.

A large part of this chapter will outline ways in which severely disabled

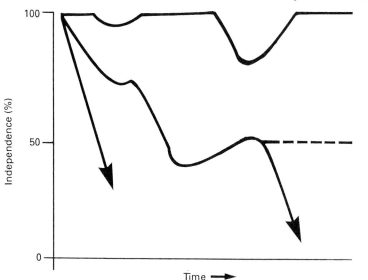

Fig. 8.1 Diagrammatic representation of the possible courses of multiple sclerosis

people with MS can be helped. They form an important group – the dominant group requiring major resources from the health and the social service departments in the age group 16–64 years. A few severely disabled people will require institutional care, depending in part on the strength of the community support services. During the course of the disease, a number of critical areas create special problems for the patients. These include learning that they have MS, the threat caused by their disease on their ability to remain at work, or adequately to play the parental role; the time when they first realize that they require an aid in order to maintain their independence; and finally for a small number, the recognition of severe disability, with the resultant acceptance of wheelchair life, dependence and occasionally the need for residential care.

The consequences on families and friends are no less great. Living with uncertainties can be very difficult, and the effects of the disease insidiously involve every area of family life. This is most marked when the disease affects intellectual function and personality. For some families – 'This is not the person I married, Doctor' – MS creates impossible pressures and many marriages break up.

DIAGNOSIS AND COUNSELLING

From an early stage, the general practitioner and consultant need to liaise in the development of support for the patients. Many consultant neurologists do not offer a follow-up service for patients with chronic neurological disease. The onus on long-term medical management is thus on the general practitioner. The national shortage of neurologists suggests that this may remain the usual practice for some time. The general practitioner has then to focus his or her attention on the 'MS family', who have the major task of supporting the person with MS, and who may previously have been unknown to the general practitioner. Patients have often found out the diagnosis for themselves, sometimes even by steaming open sealed envelopes. Others may have been told the diagnosis, and repressed this knowledge, subsequently alleging that they were never told anything at the hospital. One of us (AB) has personally experienced the uncertainty about the cause of symptoms and the relief that was felt on finally having the diagnosis confirmed.

Generally it is helpful to interview the patient and spouse together, in the presence of a social worker (provided the family agree to this) who has agreed to work with this family in the longer term. There must be prior agreement between the hospital social work service and the area office so that follow-up by the same social work team is assured. The first interview should be relatively free of details which patients are unlikely to remember after the emotional assault of learning that they have MS. Literature from the Multiple Sclerosis Society should be made available. A second interview can be arranged when patients can be encouraged to bring a list of written questions about their concerns. This is the period of maximal doubt and despair, and confidence can often be reinforced by the neurologist offering to arrange a second opinion. Some patients at this time find it helpful to be put in touch with the Multiple Sclerosis Society, but others find it distressing to be linked with patients who may be severely disabled. At this stage, the prognosis may be very uncertain, and it is reasonable to reassure patients that they may go into a remission, and for some there may be no further expression of the disease. For others, the pattern of relapse and remission will become apparent, and an unfortunate minority will progress rapidly downhill.

There is a genuine difficulty in discussing the diagnosis in patients in whom the diagnosis is uncertain. Many would agree that it is wrong to give any patient a diagnostic 'label' when there is reasonable doubt, but when it is probable that the person has MS then he or she should be told. It is to be hoped that the recent advances in diagnostic neurology will lead to an earlier diagnosis and less uncertainty. A recent survey showed that a large number of patients had not been told by their family doctors that they had MS, and most resented this. We believe patients should be told the truth about their illness as soon as the diagnosis is reasonably clear. Most patients cope with this and can be helped to do so by sympathetic and skilled listening by family doctor, social worker, friends and relatives.

For the family doctor with little experience of MS this can be a difficult period. The patient has to adjust to the new situation, as with a bereavement. The individual will feel shocked, angry and depressed, and may try to deny what has happened. This is a normal reaction and should neither be discouraged nor over-indulged. Counselling may help patients to accept their limitations. These will be both physical and psychological. A person who is mildly affected physically may be psychologically devastated, whilst someone who is severely handicapped might cope well. Adjustment can sometimes be more difficult when symptoms are mild; patients may be unsure whether to perceive themselves as normal or handicapped. Obvious physical disability may make it easier for MS sufferers to accept a new identity, but they then have to cope with the stigma of disability. Some deny their handicap, and refuse to use a stick, for example. Their subsequent staggering about can sometimes be dangerous. The doctor may be in a difficult situation, having to decide whether to encourage the individual to maintain independence for as long as possible, or to encourage the person to use aids (see also pp. 25, 33), or adopt limitations within his or her lifestyle. A balance must be found between over-accepting the disease and totally denying it, and will vary from one individual to another (Fig. 8.2).

FATIGUE

A common problem in MS is the occurrence of serious and distressing fatigue. This is a neurological phenomenon, not a psychological one, and it is often poorly understood by relatives, employers and also by health care professionals.

MS fatigue is due to an impairment of nerve conduction along demyelinated nerves, and is made worse by an increase in body temperature and by exertion. Resulting symptoms come on rapidly in patients who appear only slightly disabled initially, and both motor and sensory functions are often severely affected.

Fatigue is experienced generally as a feeling of 'flu-like' depression and specifically as an impairment of neurological function. Vision, speech, mobility, co-ordination and sensation can be badly affected even after minimal activity. Concentration and memory can also be affected by fatigue.

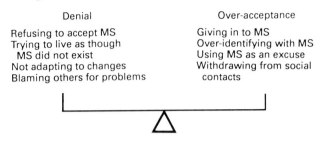

Denial   Over-acceptance

Refusing to accept MS   Giving in to MS
Trying to live as though   Over-identifying with MS
  MS did not exist   Using MS as an excuse
Not adapting to changes   Withdrawing from social
Blaming others for problems   contacts

Balanced attitude

Accepting limits, but not giving in to MS
Adapting to new ways of living, and to new roles
  at home and in the community
Living and contributing to the fullest extent possible
Creating new meanings and purposes in life

Fig. 8.2   Coming to terms with multiple sclerosis (MS). Reproduced from *Multiple Sclerosis: A Personal Exploration* (1985) by Alexander Burnfield, published by Souvenir Press, London

Typically, symptoms of fatigue occur rapidly after exercise or exertion, a hot bath, during warm weather and following infections. Normal MS symptoms are frequently made worse by exercise and warmth or even by a heavy meal. Effects are commonly at their worst in the late afternoon when the body's daily temperature cycle is at its maximum and when the person is feeling generally tired due to the increasing exertion needed to get through the day (Fig. 8.3).

Often people who have MS look physically fit, but nevertheless feel ill and are badly disabled by the fatigue. Unfortunately, fatigue is so poorly understood that some doctors may regard the patient as neurotic or as a malingerer. They may even prescribe tranquillizers or antidepressants, when what is really required is an explanation of the symptoms to both patient and family as well as reassurance and help with planning a balanced rest/exercise programme and a sensible lifestyle. Keeping as fit as possible by swimming in a cool pool will help, as will losing weight and giving up smoking if appropriate.

Fatigue can cause misunderstandings between relatives, by employers, and also by DHSS staff, and the fatigue phenomenon needs to be much better known than it is at present by all who set out to help people with MS and their families.

Hydrotherapy is seldom helpful for patients with MS because the water temperature is too high. Fatigue may, however, be markedly aggravated by failing to use aids, particularly for walking, and patients determined to

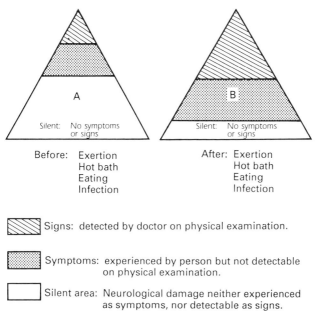

Before: Exertion
Hot bath
Eating
Infection

After: Exertion
Hot bath
Eating
Infection

Signs: detected by doctor on physical examination.

Symptoms: experienced by person but not detectable on physical examination.

Silent area: Neurological damage neither experienced as symptoms, nor detectable as signs.

Fig. 8.3 Characteristics and effects of MS fatigue, showing how symptoms are exacerbated by specific events. Reproduced from *Multiple Sclerosis: A Personal Exploration* (1985) by Alexander Burnfield, published by Souvenir Press, London

struggle on without a walking stick must realize that they may be increasing their fatigue and thus limiting their scope for leading the fullest life possible.

DOCTORS

A doctor has to combine communication and counselling skills with medical knowledge and technical expertise. This balance has not changed since the sixteenth century, when Francis Bacon wrote: 'Physicians are some of them so pleasing and conformable to the humour of the patient, as they press not the true cure of the disease; and some others are so regular in proceeding according to the art of the disease, as they respect not sufficiently the condition of the patient. Take one of a middle temper . . .'[1]

Doctors have to cope with their own feelings of inadequacy and frustration and must not take personally the anger and bitterness projected on to them by people with MS, who must live with a humiliating and frustrating disease, with loss of health, security, and changed roles within the family and working environments. The failure of quack remedies and diets can lead to anger projected on to the doctor. However, the physician can positively help patients by respect, attention, and listening. In this way the fears of the MS family can be shared and support gained by patients who feel that their doctor accepts them as fellow human beings.

One further dilemma exists for doctors trying to help people with MS in the earlier stages of the disease. Patients often dream of the miracle which will take all their disability away. The frequent remissions in this disease encourage this, and the disease sometimes 'burns out', so that a remission becomes permanent. Patients need hope, especially in the early stages. When does one stop emphasizing the hoped-for remission of tomorrow, replacing this with an insistence on coming to terms with a disease which, for that individual, is showing a progressive course, with lengthening relapses and waning remissions? This is a matter of judgement by individual doctors, but most patients' disease follows a pattern, and the local rehabilitation department can perform standardized physical and daily living assessments which document the progress of the disease. The rapid development of leg weakness or ataxia should warn patients and doctors to prepare for a wheelchair existence, and the time needed to adapt housing is such that this needs to be planned 1–2 years in advance when possible.

PREVENTION OF COMPLICATIONS

During the early course of MS habits can be acquired to prevent problems in the latter stages of the illness. Obesity, constipation, contractures and pressure sores can all be avoided or postponed with careful management. In the initial stages, a general exercise programme can be taught by physiotherapists which is designed to maintain muscle strength, prevent joint stiffness and pressure sores, and improve balance and co-ordination. Fatigue can be a major problem, and the exercise regimen must be tailored to the needs of the individual. In general, patients prefer short courses of exertion followed by short periods of rest and relaxation, and the relaxation itself may be very important. Learning this form of planned exercise provides a useful model for planning one's day in such a way that fatigue is minimized. Risks of contractures are much reduced, and patients may feel better for contributing to their own management, with a marked boost to morale. In the latter stages, physiotherapy may be combined with occupational therapy to strengthen the muscle groups needed during important movements, such as getting in and out of bed and chair, or on and off the toilet.

Although a few patients lose weight, many patients gain weight as they continue to eat enough food to maintain their previously more active life-style. Some people will be attracted to bizzare diets, but there is little evidence that any diets influence the course of the disease, except for increasing the polyunsaturated fat intake. Adequate dietary fibre is important to maintain soft stools, and patients can be advised to get into the habit of opening their bowels regularly at a similar time every day, usually after a meal. When difficulties in defaecation occur, senna the night before may stimulate the bowel. If this is unsuccessful, a local enema or suppository may be necessary. In the latter stages of the disease, constipation is frequent and bowels are best regulated by the community nursing staff. Some people are anxious to avoid manipulation of their bowel habits but the prolonged sitting on the commode/toilet may predispose to ischial pressure sores. With planning, a severely disabled person with MS (quadriplegic) can be kept at home, with the district nurse coming after breakfast to care for the pressure areas, check the catheter and clean the perineum, and assist in transfer onto commode, or perform enemata or manual evacuation if necessary. Such bowel care is usually best performed three times a week. Twice-weekly bowel care may predispose to faecal incontinence, and possibly aggravate bladder problems (Appendix 8.1).

THE MAIN CARER

From the earliest stages after diagnosis, the main carer must be supported to the full. If the carer is working, and the patient rapidly becomes severely disabled, a situation is created similar to that discussed in Chapter 5 (p. 127). A choice should be possible for the MS family. Either the carer stops working to care for the disabled partner, and the combination of attendance and mobility allowances should make this financially possible, or the family can maximize help from the local social services to enable the carer to remain at work. This option may not be available to people living in areas where there is no social services day centre, or younger disabled unit fulfilling this role.

The need for counselling has already been referred to, and the links created between the family and social worker at the time of diagnosis may be recreated at the request of the patient and family. Help may be requested by other routes. Previously mild headaches or backache may lead to presentation to the family doctor, who may give counselling or suggest help from social services.

The main carer's health is also at considerable risk. The patient may have been seeking help from the partner in walking, getting out of a chair or bed etc. Many carers put great strains on their back by bending incorrectly, particularly when helping patients out of low chairs. Social services, however, will provide a high chair with good arm rests and these can be obtained at the request of families if an occupational therapist agrees there is a need. The domiciliary physiotherapist or occupational therapist is also in a position to demonstrate how to lift people out of chairs with minimum risk to oneself.

Children may also also need help. They can grow up seeing a parent becoming increasingly disabled in front of their eyes. Some may feel they have to make every sacrifice in order to help their parents, and many seem to mature early for their years. Others can become bitter, and feel deprived and neglected, contrasting their efforts to support the parent with MS with their friends' leisure time and activities. It is important that each child should be encouraged to lead a full life, maintaining his or her own identity and independence. Some will wish to help and be prepared to make sacrifices. Others may feel repulsed and be unwilling to participate in family chores at all. They can be helped to understand the realities of the situation, and it is clearly wrong for local authorities to make plans dependent on the help of children.

Children need to understand MS in so far as they are able, and the disease should not be kept a secret from them. When major family decisions have to be made, children should be fully involved and allowed to play a part, but they should not be made to feel guilty or that they are the cause of the problem.

THE VOLUNTARY AGENCIES

It is clear that patients with MS can be helped by a vast array of professional groups, in essence deriving from the National Health Service (doctors, nurses and remedial therapists) and from the social services (social workers, community-based occupational therapists, home care workers (home helps) and care attendants). Two other sectors may be helpful; firstly the Training Commission, which, via the Disablement Resettlement Officers, may advise on all aspects of employment in relation to disabling diseases (see pp. 95, 132–3), and secondly, the voluntary sector, which is often of critical importance. Many patients derive enormous support from other MS sufferers. Apart from providing information about MS, many branches of the Multiple Sclerosis Society (Chapter 14) have voluntary workers who accumulate experience in helping people with this disease. The society has short-stay and holiday centres which it runs for its members, no matter how severely disabled, and some branches have funds available to help members with particular financial problems. Thus, a member who cannot communicate because of severe dysarthria and weakness of voice, but who could with the help of a microelectronic communicator (not available under the NHS) may be given a grant towards the cost of such equipment. Voluntary workers have occasionally helped the caring professions by attending case conferences, and may be able to help the professionals see the problems from the sufferer's point of view.

Both the Multiple Sclerosis Society and Action for Research into Multiple Sclerosis have self-help groups in which people with MS and their relatives provide counselling, emotional support and information about their disease. These groups can often provide a useful adjunct to the professional services, and at the same time it helps people with MS to feel that they can contribute to others and not just be on the receiving end, or at the bottom of the 'charity heap'. As well as helping with patient services and welfare for individuals, both these societies are major promotors of research into MS at all levels. Action for Research into Multiple Sclerosis (Chapter 14) also provides a telephone counselling service.

MOBILITY

The loss of the ability to move freely is one of the severest problems that many disabled people face. At one end of the spectrum loss of mobility (resulting from weakness, paraplegia, cerebellar ataxia or sensory loss) may lead to an inability to get in or out of bed and chair, or on and off the toilet independently. Paraplegic people have to learn to transfer themselves from their wheelchair to wherever they wish to go. When walking is possible, help may be given by suitably placed rails or grab rails, the elimination of steps or the provision of banisters.

The principles of 'environmental management' of disability – the nature and siting of the home, adapting the home for living with disability, and equipment available to facilitate personal independence – have been outlined in some detail on pp. 20–31. A few aspects of environmental management of neurological disability have been discussed on pp. 117–19, 124–6 and p. 183. Spasticity is a major problem that impedes mobility and can be helped by medical management (see below). Physiotherapy is of prime importance in the early stages, but later has to be carefully planned to avoid fatigue. It is often extremely valuable after a relapse, irrespective of whether this was associated with treatment with steroids (whether intravenously, intramuscularly or orally). Daily stretching of spastic muscles helps to relieve the stiffness and pain of spasticity, and also prevents contractures. Most health districts cannot provide physiotherapists to do this every day but the physiotherapists may be able to show family members or social service helpers how it can be done.

Physiotherapists are able to assess patients' walking ability, and advise on the probable suitability of walking aids, which may vary from a caliper to help avoid an ankle giving way, to a walking frame on wheels (rolator; Fig. 8.4). They are also able to view the rapidity of onset of fatigue, and suggest to patients when wheelchairs may be helpful for use indoors or outdoors. There may be a long period of time when a patient can utilize a wheelchair for parts of the day to avoid fatigue, but still be able to walk varying distances with or without an aid. An ataxic gait may be very difficult to alter. Some people with difficulties in plantar flexion have found the use of 'rocker' clogs helpful, although research in this field is still in its early stages.

DRIVING

Many people continue to drive for a long time. There is a legal obligation to declare to the licensing authorities if any handicap is likely to last more than 3 months. Provided that intellect, vision and reaction times are not impaired, patients can drive suitably modified cars with just one arm. Patients who are wheelchair-bound may be able to use cars modified for wheelchair users, of which a number of different types are available. Information about such vehicles can be best obtained from one of the disabled drivers' clubs. The mobility allowance can be used to finance purchase of vehicles, and details are available from Motability (see pp. 139–42). Disabled persons wishing to drive a car can be assessed at special branches of the British School of Motoring, and also at the driving assessment units at Bansted Place in Surrey and at the Princess Margaret Rose Hospital in Edinburgh (pp. 139–42). The appropriate names and addresses are provided in Chapter 14.

WHEELCHAIRS

The DHSS provides a wide variety of wheelchairs which may be self-controlled or attendant-controlled. Powered wheelchairs are available, but potential disabled users can only be referred for assessment by medical officers of the Disablement Services Authority formerly the Artificial Limb and Appliance Service in England. In Wales and Scotland this service is now incorporated in to the NHS. Only attendant-controlled powered wheelchairs

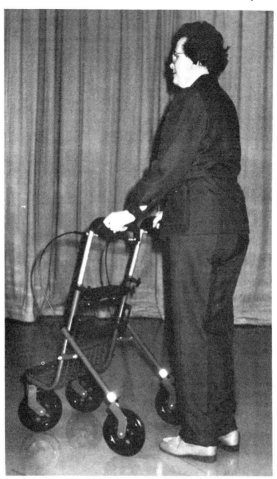

a

Fig. 8.4a–c The four-wheel walking aid 'Nova' by ETAC has cable brakes, adjustable height and seat with optional tray and basket. (Supplied in the UK by Chester Care, London, NW3 4TG)

are available at the present time for outside use through the NHS. Self-controlled powered wheelchairs or tricycles (Fig. 8.5) for outdoor use are only available privately but the mobility allowance may be used to purchase one (see Motability, and AID; pp. 139–42). Wheelchairs have to be prescribed by a doctor, and a large number of factors can influence the choice of prescription. Occupational therapists are trained to assess people's wheelchair needs, and the choice of chair is usually best left to them. General practitioners who

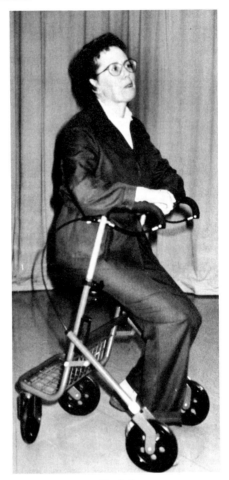

Fig. 8.4b

feel their patients require chairs can refer them directly to the occupational therapist in the local social services department. The occupational therapist will take into consideration the environment in which the chair will be used, for example, whether it needs to go into the boot of the family car, whether it will go through the door of the home, or whether the home will need the kinds of adaptations referred to on pages 124–5. Sometimes wheelchairs may be combined with commodes; special light-weight chairs may be provided by social services and may be particularly useful for the patient with prominent weakness. Some of these chairs slide over toilets.

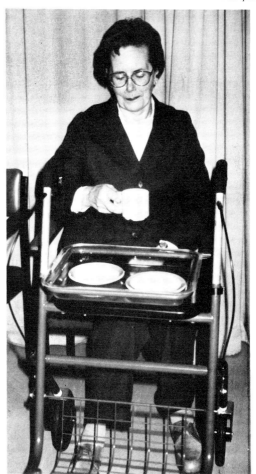

INCONTINENCE

Disorders of micturition are very distressing symptoms in MS, may be present very early in the course of the disease, and are present in almost 80% of people with established disease. Urgency, hesitancy and frequency may all be noted early in the disease, with incontinence and retention becoming more troublesome as the disease progresses. Calculi and pyelo-nephritis may be serious in the later stages.

Urinary tract infections may be inhibited with a good fluid intake, which

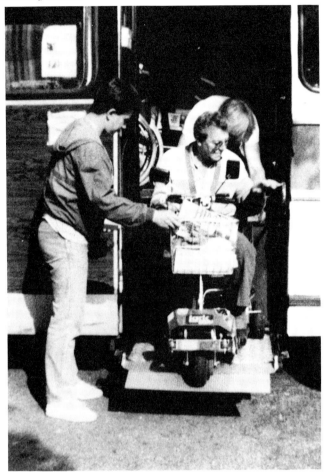

Fig. 8.5 A 55-year-old man with multiple sclerosis driving an electrically operated tricycle off the Winged Fellowship Holiday bus. This is an annual holiday which he takes by himself to give his wife some respite

can be adjusted for symptomatic relief of frequency. It is important repeatedly to exclude infections in patients with urinary symptoms, treat established infections, and prescribe prophylactic antibiotics if necessary.

Troublesome symptoms in the absence of infection warrant urological evaluation. Uninhibited detrusor muscle spasm may respond to anticholinergic drugs, or to the alpha-adrenergic blocking agent phenoxybenzamine. Results appear to be variable. Minor procedures such as urethrotomy may be helpful. Intractable retention may be helped by catheterization by intermittent urethral, long-term urethral, or suprapubic routes. Intractable incontinence may warrant a urinary diversion procedure.

The psychological consequences of disorders of micturition may outweigh their more obvious physical effects and may cause isolation due to the fear of incontinence on leaving home. This, and the importance of the physical environment, together with further details of management of disorders of micturition, are explained in Chapter 6.

SPASTICITY

Spasticity is a major problem for patients with MS. Not only can it inhibit walking, but it also may give rise to spasms which may be very painful. Spasms may also occur during transfers and may make them almost impossible. Drug treatment is usually best combined with physiotherapy, and in the ideal world tried out in hospital. Drug therapy is not without risk. The spasticity may be providing strength which the patient is using for walking, or weight-bearing during transfers. Reducing this spasticity may result in increasing weakness and a lower level of independence. In addition, in our experience patients with MS appear to be excessively susceptible to side-effects of any agents which work on the central nervous system.

Baclofen is generally agreed to be the drug of first choice, as it does not cause usually much sedation. It is most successfully used to control night cramps, and may be helpful to decrease spasticity by day. A cautious dose of 5 mg twice or thrice daily can be gently increased, with the physiotherapist giving feedback as to whether weakness is increasing, and walking improving or deteriorating. The combination of spasticity and ataxia is particularly difficult as the spasticity inhibits the ataxia, which may then worsen when spasticity is treated.

Diazepam is generally too sedative to prescribe, but may be useful at night. Dantrolene sodium acts more peripherally on the muscles, but can occasionally be useful.

PAIN

People who have MS are often told that pain is not a feature of the disease. This is not true, and pain as a symptom of MS occurs in many patients. Optic neuritis, trigeminal neuralgia and chronic spasms are well documented causes of pain, but many people also experience unpleasant burning sensations, hyperaesthesiae and similar sensory distortions, particularly in peripheral regions. These symptoms are directly related to plaques of demyelination in the central nervous system and are caused by the MS disease process.

Pain can be distressing but it is often difficult to communicate these symptoms, which are not necessarily related to physical signs. As a result they may be dismissed by doctors as 'just your MS', without further action being taken.

A large proportion of people who have MS also complain of aches and pains which may originate in muscles, joints or connective tissue. These are often indirectly caused by MS through immobility or postural abnormalities.

It is essential that pain as a symptom of MS should be recognized as soon as it occurs and investigated fully. Management will be appropriate to the individual needs of the patient, but when normal treatments fail, referral to an appropriate specialist or a pain clinic should be made.

PSYCHOLOGICAL SYMPTOMS

Traditionally euphoria has been the psychological symptom associated with MS, but evidence now suggests that severe depression is as common a problem. Euphoria certainly exists in some badly disabled patients who have associated intellectual impairment but it can mask underlying depression. Depression in these patients is thought to be directly due to the disease process and not a reactive phenomenon. Reactive depression does occur, often in the early stages of MS when a person has to grieve loss of health, status, role within the family and ultimately self-respect. In many cases, however, it is difficult to differentiate between how much depression is reactive and how much is due to the disease process, and in many patients there is probably a mixture of the two.

Even in the early stages of MS some people will experience difficulties with concentration and also with short-term memory. Emotional lability and uninhibited crying or laughing are not uncommon, and these symptoms cause patients and relatives great distress. In particular, irritability and a loss of the ability to empathize with others can cause relationship problems and breakdown, since it is seen as selfishness or as hostility and rejection.

It is important to recognize that MS commonly produces direct psychological symptoms affecting both mood and intellect, and that families with an MS member may require more than just support in coping with physical disability. Despite this many people who have MS can remain free from these distressing and humiliating psychological symptoms which often seem to be unrelated to the degree of physical handicap involved.

Individual and family counselling together with information about the disease can alleviate depression associated with the loss of physical function or role in the family. Financial help can also do much to relieve depression and emotional distress caused by loss of income, or by diminished status in the community and loss of self-respect. Some patients with persistent or severe depression will respond positively to a trial of antidepressant medication or cognitive psychotherapy. Further psychiatric treatment might usefully include family therapy at a Child and Family Guidance Centre or individually tailored behavioural therapy programmes monitored by a clinical psychologist.

SEXUAL DIFFICULTIES

Many sexual difficulties in MS are directly related to the disease process and these include varying degrees of impotence in men and orgasmic, sensory and fatigue problems in either sex. Nevertheless, sexual difficulties can also be caused or complicated by psychological or relationship factors such as depression or loss of self-respect.

A person with MS may feel unattractive to others and this can lead either to withdrawal from sexual or social relationships, or to an attempt to compensate by being sexually demanding.

Where anger is a major feature of relationships, as is so often the case when one person is dependent on another, then a sexual relationship will often be very difficult. Cultural factors play a large part in the way that people adjust to sexual difficulties so an overall assessment of the problem must include an appreciation of the person concerned physically, psychologically and socially.

Unfortunately, people who have MS are far too often told: 'It is your MS. You should forget about sex – you will have to live with the situation.' This is not a justified response since a great deal can be done through counselling or by providing information and education to both partners. Many people can manage to learn new sexual behaviours providing that they are open and honest with each other and able to experiment, for instance with penile prostheses. It will sometimes be necessary to get away from an obsession with sexual intercourse in order to find new and more appropriate methods of showing sexual expression. Counselling in this area requires special skills and understanding by all health care professionals. A useful organization both for disabled people with sexual problems and for professionals is Sexual and Personal Relationships of the Disabled (SPOD).

PREGNANCY

Although women with MS commonly report a relapse or exacerbation of symptoms once a baby is born, there is no evidence that the disease will be made worse in the long term by pregnancies. There is also no evidence that the contraceptive pill will do any harm to people who have MS and sensible family planning is of paramount importance if one partner has the disease.

SPEECH AND COMMUNICATION

Impaired speech in MS is usually due to weakness, poor control of breathing, dysarthria, or a combination of these. Communication can be helped by supporting the spine and neck of a weak patient in his or her chair or wheelchair. The speech therapist is able to help patients co-ordinate their breathing with their talking, and with their articulation. Patients who fatigue easily will notice that fatigue affects their speech, and the speech therapist is able to help patients plan their day so that the voice does not fatigue too early. The tense patient may be taught relaxation techniques to enhance speech. The severely speech-disabled patient may be able to use a communicator, although the less expensive communicators may be unsuitable for patients without a useful hand. More recently, microprocessor-controlled devices have come into use, although their price is out of the range of the NHS and most patients. Funding for such devices, however, can often be obtained from local voluntary agencies such as the Lions or Round Table. Sometimes the Multiple Sclerosis Society may be able to help financially.

A different aspect of communication is that of being able to get help in an emergency. Telephones may be adapted for ease of use, and externally sounding alarms installed. The system which works very satisfactorily in Harrow is the Harrow Helpline: the individual at risk wears a radio pendant around the neck. When the emergency button on either the pendant or telephone is pressed the person can speak to the control centre staff who summon appropriate help. Many similar schemes operate in different parts of the country.

SUPPORT FOR THE SEVERELY DISABLED PERSON

Even very severely disabled people with MS can be maintained in the community if that is their wish (see Appendix 8.1). The cementing of the links

Table 8.1   Funding of community support for severely disabled persons

Agency	Financial consequences	
	Capital	Revenue
Health	Wheelchairs Mattresses Beds Environmental control	Hire of expensive bed, e.g. with low air loss Provision of nursing care (bladder, bowels) Incontinence service Domiciliary physiotherapist District dental officer Community dietitian
Social services	Simple aids Major aids, e.g. electric chairs, elevators/stair lift etc.	Community-based occupational therapy Social worker (e.g. counselling) Home care service (home help) Care Attendant
Either service	Hoists	Assisting washing, feeding, transfers, being there when needed
Local authority	Provision of house or adapting house or garden (e.g. steps, drive etc.)	Maintenance of property if owned by council

between the hospital and community health services and the social services is usually best done by a case conference (see pp. 123–4).

The philosophy of the social services is critical, as outlined in Chapter 13. Community support becomes progressively more difficult or sometimes impossible, irrespective of maximal community support, in the presence of withdrawal of support from carer(s), severe intellectual deterioration, intractable extrapyramidal symptoms, intractable faecal incontinence or the necessity for tube-feeding. Table 8.1 outlines the responsibilities of the caring agencies to provide this support. Some authorities are backward in providing these services, and many health authorities have not planned sufficiently for the capital costs of maintaining severely disabled people in the community. Where the caring agencies work together, severely disabled people can be supported at home with dignity. Where patients do not wish to remain at home, residential care can be arranged in a younger disabled unit, Cheshire Home, or long-stay hospital, possibly in the private sector, such as the Royal Hospital and Home, Putney (Chapter 14).

The importance of day support is emphasized on pp. 127–8 and 256–7. The provision of an occupational therapist at such a centre helps good liaison with the health rehabilitation departments and promotes common therapeutic aims. Such day centre support may be utilized once per month, or five days a week according to need and available resources. Some younger disabled units fill this role and successfully meet physical, social and emotional needs in this way.

Holiday relief may be necessary to provide a break for the caring relative (Fig. 8.5), and sometimes even for the professional carers. Where there are no specific medical needs, this can be provided by the social services, sometimes using charities such as the Winged Fellowship Trust (Chapter 14) and occasionally financial help may be given by the Multiple Sclerosis Society. Where there is a necessity for re-evaluation of physical needs (e.g. increasing disability following a relapse of MS) this may be best performed in a rehabilitation ward, or a younger disabled unit.

Many people successfully overcome their physical disability until, in older age, they develop multiple handicaps. This is discussed in Chapter 7, and the best service is likely to be provided by the local department of geriatric medicine, unless services are available elsewhere in the district to provide hospital, rehabilitation and social support in their advancing years.

THE END-STAGES

Where the family unit has been maintained, strains universally appear within it. The strains on the main carer, usually the spouse, have been discussed above. Cantrell et al[2] found only 1 out of 100 families affected by a very severely handicapped person where the main helper was 'healthy and problem-free'. Risk factors for the breakdown of the support network[3] are both intrinsic (within the client) and extrinsic (within the family, home, or community) – see Table 8.2.

It is critical to determine the individual's assets – those hidden resources which, if developed, will enable that person to lead the fullest life possible. Anything which stimulates interest or enthusiasm may give a huge boost to morale.

As in all incurable illnesses, the end will come one day, albeit for many people with MS, in old age. Death may not necessarily be related to MS as many people with this disease have a normal life span and die of something else.

People have the right to express views about where and how they die, and these should be respected if possible. Frank discussions with a professional

Table 8.2 Intrinsic and extrinsic factors contributing to the breakdown of the support network of the multiple sclerosis sufferer[3]

Intrinsic problems

Increasing paralysis or sensory loss
Intellectual or speech defects
Personality change (particularly loss of humour)
Fatigue
Loss of confidence (e.g. after a fall, incontinence)
Boredom – loss of meaning to life
Infections
Drug or alcohol abuse
Pressure sores

Extrinsic problems

Lack of recuperation time (caring for 24 hours/day)
Denial of problems
Conflict of care, e.g. with work
Isolation
Poverty
Ill health (backache, hypertension)
Fatigue (heavy load getting heavier)
Role change
Sexual change
Sexual frustration
Loss of future – living with no hope of a cure

who has a good rapport with the individual – often the general practitioner – may enable policies to be formulated for the management of acute inter-current medical conditions.

CONCLUSIONS

There are many ways in which those who live with MS may be helped. Major strains can be taken away from the main carer, but some families refuse all offers of help, particularly when the spouse feels that he or she alone ought to care for the loved one. Monitoring these families often fails unless health districts or local authorities set up careful services. Nevertheless, much can be done, and people with MS should never be told: 'You have multiple sclerosis, and there is no treatment. We cannot help you.' Instead we can say: 'Although at the present time there is no known cure for the disease, we will support you and your family through all stages of your illness.'

REFERENCES

1. Bacon F. (1972), Essay XXX: of regiment of health, *Modern Ed.*, London, J. M. Dent.
2. Cantrell T., Dawson J., Glastonbury G. (1983), *Prisoners of Handicap – A study of Dependency in Young Physically Disabled People and the Families of People upon whom they Rely*, Southampton University, Rehabilitation Unit.
3. DHSS (1982), Multiple sclerosis, *Demonstration Centres in Rehabilitation Newsletter*; 29: 1–39.

FURTHER READING

Anonymous (1983), Treatment of multiple sclerosis, *Lancet*; 1: 909–10.

Burnfield A. (1984), Doctor–patient dilemmas in multiple sclerosis, *J. Med. Ethics*; 1: 21–6.

Burnfield A. (1985), *Multiple Sclerosis: A Personal Exploration*, Human Horizons Series, London, Souvenir Press.

Burnfield A., Burnfield F. (1978), Common psychological problems in multiple sclerosis, *Br. Med. J.*; 1: 1193–4.

Langton-Hewer R. (1980), Multiple sclerosis: management and rehabilitation, *Int. Rehab. Med.*; 2: 116–25.

Simons A. E. F. (1984), *Psychological and Social Aspects of Multiple Sclerosis*, London, William Heinemann Medical Books.

Symposium on Multiple Sclerosis (1982), *Physiotherapy*; 68: 144–5.

Appendix 8.1

Case histories

Two case histories illustrate the ability to maintain severely disabled individuals at home in spite of the severity of their disability, provided there is a desire on the part of the individual to be at home, and of the caring professions to support him or her in that desire. The histories are portrayed through the eyes of the district nurses who have known and supported both individuals for many years.

Few patients with multiple sclerosis become so extremely dependent, but the histories illustrate how some of the handicaps of a severely disabled individual can be overcome so that the person can maintain a meaningful and dignified life within the community.

Case history 1

Mrs X is a 41-year-old divorcee with multiple sclerosis, and effectively tetraplegic. She lives with her 13-year-old daughter. Known to the district nurses for 12 years, her needs had gradually increased as her disease progressed until nursing visits were numbering 4 per 24 hours. The morning visit was the most time-consuming, lasting in excess of 2 hours. Actual nursing care consisted of a daily blanket bath, catheter and bowel care, and treatment of a deep pressure sore – in all taking about 45 minutes. The nurses then needed to hoist her into her wheelchair and position her until comfortable (in itself a 20 minute exercise) and transport her downstairs in the lift installed by social services. They would then prepare and give her her breakfast. Interspersed with all this they fed the cat, paid the milkman, and answered the telephone or door as necessary.

A return visit in the afternoon was made to put her on her bed for a rest. Her young daughter would get her up on return from school and the district nurses would put her back to bed in the evening, returning at around 03.00 h to turn her and give her a drink. Home helps cooked lunch for her and left sandwiches for supper.

With the aim of keeping this small family unit intact, and even more importantly, relieving the strain on the young daughter, social services and health services agreed to jointly fund care attendant support. The teaching role of the district nurse was utilized to train this new team of carers to use the electric hoist and handle the patient safely, since she was now totally dependent. Once the carers were confident and working to a carefully planned timetable, their input enabled the nursing service to reduce the morning visit to half an hour and eliminate the second and third visits. The district night nurse continued to visit at 03.00 h to reposition her and give her a drink.

The objective of keeping mother and daughter together in their own home, as they both desperately wanted, was achieved. The hourly input of the district nursing ser‑vice was approximately halved.

Case history 2

Mrs Z is a 54-year-old lady suffering from multiple sclerosis with onset of symptoms about 20 years ago. She lived with her husband, but there were no children. Her father came to live with them about that time 'for her to look after him' after the death of his wife.

She first became known to the district nursing service 14 years ago. As her physical condition deteriorated her husband took on the caring role until he was forced to give up work 11 years ago on the grounds of ill health. District nursing input then increased until her husband's admission to hospital 6 years later with chronic bronchitis, when she too was admitted as a 'social admission'. Following her husband's discharge 3 months later, district nurses undertook all her nursing care, by which time Mrs Z was unable to stand and suffered severe muscle spasms. Six months later her husband died suddenly from a coronary thrombosis, but by then her condition had improved slightly and she was able to do some cooking and light housework from her wheelchair. However, this remission was short-lived and within a year of her husband's death she became incontinent of urine and very depressed, being more and more dependent on help from the district nurse.

Two years ago she sustained a pathological fractures (from osteomalacia) of the left neck of femur. Her father, who was now in his late 80s and profoundly deaf, provided an element of support (he could at least make her cups of tea) but his constant fussing over her, compounded by his extreme deafness, became a burden to her and the relationship between them deteriorated to the extent that violent incidents between them were reported. His admission to hospital with pneumonia precipitated a crisis necessitating her admission as well 'because she was totally dependent and could not remain at home unsupported'.

When her father's condition had improved a case conference was convened with medical, nursing, and social work representatives – both hospital and community – present for both father and daughter (see also pp. 123–5). Mrs Z had already spent an unhappy trial period in a young disabled unit and was now adamant that she wanted to return to her own home. It was therefore planned to discharge her home on a 2-week trial basis before the discharge of her father. This decision was made on the basis that the house belonged to her and not to him.

With total co-operation between district nursing and social services a careful timetable was drawn up planning her care over 24 hours. Downstairs accommodation in her semi-detached house had already been adapted long before her admission to hospital, and an electric hoist had been installed by social services over her bed at the far end of the through lounge. A suitable hospital-type bed was, however, purchased for her by health services as her own new divan bed was quite unsuitable since it was too low, resulting in back strain for the nursing staff prior to her admission. The provision of a Buxton chair by social services was successful in overcoming her fear, both real and imaginary, of sliding out of her wheelchair.

Because of her precarious physical condition, all nursing care was undertaken by trained nurses – normally the district nursing sister assisted by one of her team. Home care workers came to sit Mrs Z up and give her breakfast each morning before the nursing staff arrived, and returned to cook and feed her lunch and tea in addition to the usual household tasks required of them. District nurses put her back to bed in the afternoon, as by this time she was always very tired, but further visits were made during the evening and around 02.00 h to reposition her and give her a drink.

Social services had previously installed a front door entry telephone with automatic release, which gave Mrs Z the facility to admit her visitors when she was alone. Regular visits from her general practitioner each week were a great morale boost, and her health visitor called each week for a chat.

During her trial period at home her father suddenly died while still in hospital. This in fact resolved a potential problem and her planned re-admission to hospital did not take place. She is now extremely happy at home and will be able to remain there for the foreseeable future. When the time comes it should be possible for her to die in her own home with the additional support of care attendants and extra night nursing.

9

Helping parents of children with cancer

Peter Maguire and Pat Morris Jones

INTRODUCTION

Many parents will not have realized that the symptoms complained of by their child are due to a serious and life-threatening illness. Instead, they may have interpreted the illness as due to a virus or to 'growing pains'. So the first task is to help parents make the transition from a perception of their child as having a minor illness to acknowledging that he or she has a cancer. The aim is to help them assimilate the bad news without them becoming hopeless about their child's long-term prospects.

BREAKING THE NEWS

It will usually be the haematologist or paediatrician who informs the parents. Whenever possible both parents should be present when the news is given. Each parent may only remember a proportion of what was said because of the emotional shock caused by the information. They can then discuss between them what was said and so recall much more. Sharing this time of crisis should also enable them to give each other support. Involving both parents may indicate to the clinician that there are already problems between the couple which could hinder their ability to adapt.

It is important to begin by firing a 'warning shot' to give the parents an indication that what they are to be told is serious. This allows them time to prepare themselves psychologically.

Doctor: I thought I should talk to you both about Tommy's condition straight away.

Mother: Oh! What is it?

Doctor: I am afraid that it has turned out to be much more serious than we thought originally. It isn't, I am afraid, anaemia.

Father: What do you mean, more serious?

Doctor: It's turned out to be a problem with how he is forming his blood cells.

Mother: How do you mean?

Doctor: Well, I have to tell you that he has a cancer of the blood-forming cells. I want to refer him to a specialist centre for treatment.

When the news has been conveyed it is essential that parents should be allowed time to assimilate it. The temptation to soften the blow by suggesting: 'It is not as bad as it sounds' or saying: 'Everything is going to be all right' should be resisted. This promotes denial and leads to bitterness when parents realize the gravity of the child's illness.

However well the information is conveyed it will inevitably distress the parents and may be misunderstood. The clinician undertaking the treatment should explore how information has affected the parents and encourage them to express any concerns.

Doctor: Dr Allen has told you that Tommy has a cancer of the blood?

Mother: What do you mean a cancer of the blood?

Doctor: Well, it's called leukaemia. His white blood cells, which are essential to his fighting infections, are not forming properly. He is also not forming enough cells to stop bleeding. That's why he's been haemorrhaging. I am sorry to have to confirm this. How are you feeling?

Father: It's a terrible blow to us. Our local hospital initially suggested it was some kind of anaemia. We hoped it was and nothing more serious. It's hard for us to think that he might not be here for very much longer.

Doctor: Why do you say that?

Father: Cancer, even cancer of the blood, usually means a death sentence, doesn't it?

Doctor: No, it doesn't.

Father: How do you mean?

Doctor: Well, while he has a form of cancer, the good news is that we can get it under control and he could do well in the longer term.

Father: How do you mean, well?

Doctor: I think there is a good chance that we might be able to cure him. However we won't be able to tell this for some time.

Mother: Do you mean there's a chance then?

Doctor: I honestly think there is but, of course, I can't guarantee it. I'm sure
    we'll get him into remission. Then we'll have to see how he gets on.
    Are there any other questions you would like to ask?
Mother: No, I don't think so at the moment. There is so much to take in.
Father: No, I think that's all now.
Doctor: Well, I can see that it has been quite a shock. If you do have any
    further questions over the next few days, please do get back to me.
    I'll do my best to see you and answer them. It is obviously going to
    be hard for you to take all of this in. But the good news is that I
    think we should be able to do something for him. Are there any
    other concerns you would like to raise?
Mother: No, I don't think so.
Father: No.
Doctor: OK. Would you like to come and see me in a week's time so I can
    give you an update on to what's happening?
Mother: Yes.

The clinican was honest about the child's situation but left the parents
with genuine hope that something can be done. Words were used to mirror
the expectation of the likely outcome and the temptation to mislead parents
that their child's outlook was better than was thought was resisted.

If the assessment of the prognosis of the cancer was poor, words would
have been used like: 'We hope that we will be able to control his disease in
the short term'. Parents are more likely to adapt if they are given a realistic
appraisal of their child's prognosis.

However well the bad news is broken and confirmed, most parents feel
devastated. Such occasions may not be the best time to give them much
more information about their child's illness. They will not register much of
it however carefully it is given. Consequently it is valuable to offer them a
further appointment within a few days as it is usually essential to begin treating the cancer as soon as possible; treatment options should be discussed
honestly and parents warned about likely adverse effects, including possible
dangers. If the child is to be entered into a clinical trial the basis of the trial
should be explained and the known advantages and disadvantages of the different treatments discussed before seeking the parents' consent.

MONITORING REACTIONS

When parents are next seen by the clinician it is important to monitor how
they have reacted to their child's illness and initial treatment. This can be

done by asking each parent in turn how he or she has been affected by hearing that the child has cancer. It is useful to ask both parents whether at any stage since diagnosis they have felt especially low, miserable or tense and anxious. Parents should also be asked whether they understood what was said to them about their child's illness and treatment. This enquiry should reveal whether they have developed any misconceptions and these should be explored, clarified and corrected.

Most parents are likely to be distressed in this period after diagnosis. It is useful to establish the nature and extent of any anxiety and depression; this will provide a baseline measure against which to judge later adaptation. It also shows an interest in how parents are faring and will encourage them to disclose subsequent problems.

KEY QUESTIONS

Parents have to resolve several critical questions if they are to adapt psychologically. So the clinician, nurse or social worker needs to check how they are handling these questions within the first few weeks of diagnosis.

Why our child?

Cancer is rare in childhood and there are still no adequate scientific theories to account for its development. Yet parents are often desperate to find an explanation and may fill the vacuum with unhelpful theories, as the following example illustrates.

> A young mother had been a staunch Roman Catholic. However, she was pressed to use a contraceptive pill by her husband despite contrary advice from her priest. She took the pill for 3 years and then both she and her husband decided that they wanted another baby. She therefore stopped the pill with his agreement and soon became pregnant. The pregnancy was uneventful and the child, a girl, appeared to be developing normally. However, she then developed leukaemia and the mother became convinced despite argument that she was being punished by God for going against the priest's advice. She became severely depressed and suicidal.

Parents may wrongly implicate recent stresses as a cause, for example, a bereavement or divorce. They may blame themselves for having transmitted the stress to the child and for not having coped more effectively. Alternatively a parent may blame the partner and become consumed with bitterness. Either parent may worry that the illness has been passed on by them through a gene or viral infection. Radiation from nuclear power stations is now considered a possible aetiological factor, so parents may blame themselves for living near a power station.

To pick up unhelpful theories both parents should be asked: 'Why do *you* think your child has got cancer?' and the reasons for their answers explored.

Should we treat our child as normal?

The child could die within the next few years, possibly from exposure to measles or chickenpox when immunosuppressed from chemotherapy. So, should the child be expected to go to school, socialize as usual with peers and be subject to normal discipline? There is a strong risk that some parents will keep the child from school unnecessarily, prevent him or her from playing with friends and over-protect and indulge him or her. Each parent should be asked: 'Is he/she back at school yet?', 'Does he/she see as much of his/her friends as he/she used to?', 'Has there been any change in the way you discipline him/her?' and 'How much do you expect him/her to do for him/ herself?' When the replies suggest problems with behaviour or school attendance it is useful to liaise with the school directly.

Will our child survive?

While most cancers will be eradicated by initial treatment parents will obviously be concerned about the child's eventual prognosis. Even with bio- logical indicators of longer-term response there will still be much uncer- tainty and this should be acknowledged by the clinician. The doctor should then discuss markers that will indicate that the child could be experiencing a relapse, for example, large swollen glands (as in lymphoma). It also helps if parents are given direct access so that any possible relapse can be discussed with the doctor quickly and appropriate action can be taken. Meanwhile the parents should be asked how often they would like to review progress, since few will abuse this invitation.

Father: What are his chances?
Clinician: The trouble is, I don't know at this point. I think they could be good but I can't be certain.
Father: Surely you can give me a better estimate than that?
Clinician: I'd like to and it is good that he is still in remission. I see no reason why he shouldn't stay well – and the longer it goes the better he should do. In the meantime we'll keep an eye on him.
Father: That's fine. I presume we can get in touch with you between times if there are any problems.

Clinician: It's most important that you should feel able to do that. If there's any change in his health that concerns you or that you're not sure about, for goodness sake ring me or one of my team directly.

What can we do?

Parents may feel helpless because they believe that they can do nothing to contribute to their child's recovery. Others may be more positive and seek out as much information as they can to ensure their child gets optimal treatment. They may even look to alternative cancer therapies and pursue the use of purgation and special diets. They may help with fund-raising to improve the chances of a cure being found (e.g. for Leukaemia Research Fund; see Chapter 14).

It is important to identify whether parents are taking an active or helpless stance by asking: 'Do you think there is anything you can do to combat your child's illness?' When a parent is looking to alternative therapies to complement conventional ones this should be encouraged unless it could become an over-riding obsession and cause serious problems. The 'pros and cons' of alternative therapies should then be discussed in a non-judgemental way.

What will treatment be like?

The treatments used to combat cancer in children (like radiotherapy and chemotherapy) have to be potent in order to destroy the cancer cells. However they can destroy normal tissue as well and cause unpleasant adverse effects like hair loss, nausea, vomiting and mouth ulcers; parents should be warned about this. While they may then imagine the worst they should soon realize that the effects are not as bad as they had forecast and they will adjust better. If the doctor insists on using euphemisms – such as: 'Even if your daughter is sick it'll only be a little sickness' – parents may become angry and bitter because they were misled about the seriousness of the adverse effects. Moreover they will distrust statements made by other doctors and this could become crucial if there are crises in the child's illness. Parents can be reassured if they are told that if their child does experience adverse effects they should contact the doctor or one of the team directly, so that the adverse affects can be explored and appropriate action taken.

How do we maintain a balance?

For most parents their child's illness will become an over-riding concern in the first few months after diagnosis. They may then neglect each other's needs and the needs of other children. This is particularly likely if the illness follows a stormy and unpredictable course. Mothers especially can become distanced from the rest of the family because they spend all their time with the sick child. This is often inadvertently encouraged by the treatment centre because of the current philosophy of expecting parents to be with their child in hospital. The parents may have too little time away from the situation and find that their physical and emotional resources are being depleted. They may also discover that other members of the family are feeling resentful and neglected. It is important to discuss this issue and encourage parents to maintain as good a balance as possible despite the burden of coping with a sick child and regular visits to hospital.

Should we be open about it?

Adaptation is facilitated within the family by telling a child who is old enough to understand what is wrong – that is, that he or she has a serious disease but it can be treated. This will then make sense of the treatments and follow-up which must be endured. Siblings should also be told, otherwise they may be bewildered and upset by changes in their parents and the affected child. So it is useful to enquire of the patients: 'Have you been able to tell Tommy what is wrong?' and to follow this up according to the response with 'How has he taken it' or 'Why haven't you told him?'

Openness with close friends and relatives is also associated with a better longer-term adjustment. Parents should be asked: 'Have you been able to tell your close relatives and friends?' and their responses should be explored accordingly: 'How did they react?' or 'What has held you back?'

Doctor: So, you have only told one friend, why is that?
Father: That was bad enough. He made me feel that Tommy had leprosy. He seems to feel that his children could catch it in some way.

Parents also have to decide how open they should be with each other about their concerns. Too little sharing can provoke resentment and too much can mean that neither parent gets any respite. Ideally, parents will be open with each other but will spread the load by confiding in others. This can be assessed by asking: 'Have you been able to be open with each other?' Disagreement between a couple about how open they should be with each other, their children or others can provoke much friction and should be resolved if possible.

How will others react?

When close relatives and friends realize that the family have a sick child they will usually do their utmost to provide support because they believe that the crisis will be resolved soon. When they realize that they are confronted by a chronic illness they may find it difficult to continue to provide support. They are not sure what they can discuss with safety. For example, if they ask how the child is doing now they may learn that the child is having very un-pleasant side-effects from the treatment or has relapsed. Moreover the parents are unlikely to say anything positive in the first few months because the child's prognosis is still uncertain. Consequently, some relatives and friends telephone or visit less and even avoid any contact. The family of the sick child may thus become increasingly isolated and this will make them more vulnerable psychologically because support is an important buffer against the risk of psychiatric breakdown.

It is important to emphasize to parents the value of maintaining contacts with friends and relatives and help them anticipate possible difficulties in these relationships and resolve them. Problems of isolation can also be mini-mized by encouraging parents to talk informally with other parents.

PRACTICAL PROBLEMS

Most children with cancer are treated in regional centres located a consider-able distance from the family's home. Regular travel to these centres can create problems. Journeys may prove too costly and parents may find it diffi-cult to get time off work. There is then a danger that one parent, usually the mother, will bear the brunt of visiting and spend most of her time with the sick child. So it is useful to discuss how parents plan to manage the burden of visiting and to encourage both partners to share the load when possible. It is important to stress that parents are entitled to time off and must not feel they should visit all the time. They can also be told that financial help is available if they need it.

PSYCHIATRIC MORBIDITY

However well the doctors try to inform the parents about the child's cancer and treatment and help them resolve these formidable questions a propor-tion of parents will fail to cope and develop psychiatric problems. Thus in one study of 60 families who were followed up from the time their child was first diagnosed at a major treatment centre in Manchester, 25% of mothers had an anxiety state 12 to 18 months later compared with 5% of mothers of children who were treated during the same period for minor illnesses.[1] This accorded with the high levels of anxiety noted by Tiller et al (42%)[2] and Marten et al (45%),[3] studying smaller groups. Similarly, studies by Magni et al[4] and Peck[5] also found an excess of anxiety in mothers of children with cancer compared with control groups. Thus it seems reasonable to conclude that, despite the small samples employed and the differences in methodology, at least 1 in 5 mothers in the first year or two after diagnosis will develop an anxiety state which is severe enough to warrant help. This represents a fivefold increase in relative risk compared with control groups.

In the study carried out in Manchester, 23% of mothers had a depressive illness at the 12- to 18-month follow-up point compared with only 7% in a control group.[1] This represented a threefold increase in relative risk. Marten et al[3] and Tiller et al[2] also reported higher rates of depression (38% and 38% respectively). Overall, between 1 in 4 and 1 in 3 mothers who have a child being treated for cancer will show evidence of an anxiety state and/or depression 12 to 18 months after treatment.

While fathers appear less at risk of psychiatric morbidity some may develop anxiety and/or depression.

Sexual problems

One-fifth of mothers in the Manchester study who had an enjoyable sex life before the diagnosis of their child's illness experienced a marked deterioration in the follow-up period compared with 8% in the control groups.[1] Many mothers explained this on the grounds that they had no right to enjoy themselves while their child was so ill. Others explained their loss of libido in relation to continued anxiety, depression or both. In some instances it stemmed from their allowing the child into the marriage bed because the child had behaviour tantrums if left alone.

Longer-term psychological morbidity

As yet there has been no adequate long-term follow-up of parents of children with cancer, therefore it is not known what happens to psychiatric morbidity over time.

INTERVENTION

Use of specialist nurses and social workers

Many centres have appointed specialist nurses or social workers, often through the agency of charities like the Malcolm Sargeant Fund or local authorities. They have done so in the hope that psychological morbidity would be prevented if parents were visited regularly and given practical advice, information and emotional support. The scheme described by Michelutte and her colleagues in 1981[1] typifies this approach. A specialist paediatric nurse visited all newly diagnosed children and their families shortly after discharge home and once the cancer had been brought into remission. She also attempted to follow-up all children who were terminally ill. This scheme was evaluated by assesssing families 2 months and 6 to 11 months after diagnosis. A total of 89% of those she saw found her visits useful but more objective measures showed no change. Those who were visited showed as much depression and distress as parents who had not been visited. Nor was there any difference between the overall functioning of visited and non-visited families. This failure of simple advice, information and emotional support to prevent psychological morbidity accords with the findings of studies of counselling of adult cancer patients.[7,8] It emphasizes the need for further evaluation of the role and impact of specialist nurses and social workers within the area of childhood leukaemia.

When parents were asked about the impact of the nurse they indicated that she needed more training in specific counselling skills. Morrow et al[9] also found that over half of the parents of children with cancer they studied felt that they would have benefited from more counselling. Unfortunately, the definition of 'counselling' was not clarified in either of these studies, so it is not clear what parents were seeking. It is probable that they would welcome active interventions like being taught anxiety management techniques (such as relaxation or meditation) rather than just talking about problems. Such interventions should be tested to evaluate whether they can markedly reduce anxiety and depression in parents. Alternatively it may be naive to expect to prevent problems when parents are facing such uncertainty and trying to resolve several major questions.

Use of groups

Many centres have set up support groups in the belief that they could help parents. This is an attractive solution since a specialist worker can try and help several parents at once and parents can benefit from talking to each other. Such groups should reduce isolation, provide relevant information, foster emotional support and facilitate adaptation by encouraging parents to share relevant experiences, express feelings, discuss specific concerns and problems and then explore and monitor attempts to resolve them. Such groups may utilize professional advice and invite input about particular themes, for example, the latest development in treatment.

Many doctors still worry that such groups cause more harm than good, especially when the parents have children with different prognoses and a child with a poor prognosis dies. Until there is a proper evaluation of the short- and longer-term effects of such groups it is difficult to refute this charge. Meanwhile, Adams[10] has indicated that if groups are to be helpful they must be controlled by leaders who can set firm limits about what can and cannot be discussed or disclosed and who are willing to moderate discussion. Group leaders should also have a good knowledge of family and group dynamics. Even if these criteria are satisfied there is no guarantee that all parents will be helped. Studies are needed, therefore, to confirm that such leadership is associated with positive outcomes.

A major limitation to support groups[11] is that those who most need support do not attend them; a survey is needed of the long-term outcome of attenders and non-attenders to examine this issue. Moreover some parents who become involved only do so for a short time; only a small proportion of all parents attend support groups consistently over time.

Self-help

Parents of a child with cancer have a unique advantage over most professionals in that they have experienced what it is like to have a child with such an illness and are aware of the effects of treatment. Some centres have utilized this by asking parents to advise and support other parents of newly diagnosed children or parents facing particular problems. Meeting with a parent who had problems in adapting but subsequently coped can be encouraging to a parent who is still struggling to overcome the main obstacles. It can reduce feelings of isolation and alienation[12] and make parents feel it is legitimate to discuss and express concerns. It also affords a model of possible coping strategies. However, the use of volunteers carries certain dangers: they may have volunteered to resolve their own problems. This could lead them to talk only about their own experiences rather than listen to their clients. Parents may have volunteered because they are confident that they will be able to cope with any eventuality, including their child's death. Such parents may find it hard to tolerate a parent who is struggling to cope and they may impose their own modes of coping as the only way forward. They may also be induced into the role of the strong helping the weak.

Such difficulties can be avoided if parents who volunteer are carefully selected and trained in listening and counselling skills.[13] Even so, several major questions remain unresolved. What are the selection criteria which work best? What is the best method of training volunteers so that they avoid harming parents and yet are not perceived as too professional? How long can volunteers work without becoming too involved or adversely affected by it? Experience in some centres has suggested that volunteers should work for only 2 years before contributing to self-help organizations in a more administrative or social capacity. What support and supervision do such volunteers need? Will they accept it? It remains to be seen how many volunteers would allow an assessment of their work.

HELPING THOSE AT RISK

Resources could be used most efficiently if parents who were to develop problems could be identified early. Kaplan et al[14] found some identifiable factors which predicted those parents who failed to cope. These included unrealistic expectations of cure, an unwillingness to discuss the illness or share feelings within the family, differences in parents' ways of coping, and one parent bearing a disproportionate burden of the illness and treatment. Similarly, women who have no one they can confide in but who avoid over-burdening any one person and so have no proper confidant; parents whose child has severe adverse effects due to treatment; and those with marked restriction of social and leisure activities are more at risk.

While these factors seem promising for the prediction of those at risk, they need rigorous testing within prospective studies to assess whether targeting such parents and intervening identifies those at risk and reduces psychological and social morbidity.

Work by Fife[15] has suggested that certain behaviours may be difficult to change even if they are discovered early on in treatment. The author tried to prevent mothers becoming over-protective through intervention. In the client-centred intervention she used a non-directive approach to help mothers consider alternative ways of relating to the child and the consequence of each option. In an alternative method she used a behavioural approach and set parents clear goals and tasks. Both interventions had mixed results, with some parents reducing their over-protection but others becoming more protective. These data emphasize the need for careful controlled studies of interventions designed to prevent morbidity and promote rehabilitation.

The attitude of 'at risk' parents to the offer of help could be crucial. They may believe that they are coping well and resent the suggestion that they require help. Consequently, only a small proportion of 'at risk' parents may co-operate with early intervention. Studies need to be carried out to determine whether aftercare which limits itself to those at risk is as effective as the monitoring of all parents' progress.

EARLY DETECTION

As with women after mastectomy, the psychological morbidity usually remains hidden and the reasons for this are similar (see Chapter 10). Training which includes the use of audiotape recording of practice interviews, feedback and discussion with a tutor has proved effective in helping specialist nurses improve their ability to monitor cancer patients and detect most of the problems that present.[7] Such improvement has also been found when ward nurses are given similar training.[16] It should be possible to extend such monitoring in the community by training health visitors and district nurses in these skills, but attempts to involve health visitors in the aftercare of children with leukaemia have failed. They felt uneasy at being involved in the care of children with cancer. Despite a brief training they considered that they lacked the necessary counselling and assessment skills. They felt overburdened with other tasks and tended to avoid families with a child suffering from cancer. Thus the aftercare of children with cancer is likely to remain in the domain of specialist nurses and social workers for the present time.

PSYCHOLOGICAL INTERVENTION

Any parents found to have an anxiety state, depressive illness, sexual problem or marital problem should be referred to their general practitioner in the first instance. Conventional psychological and psychiatric treatments should then be used and a proportion of parents are likely to improve with that help alone. However, others will continue to have problems and should then be referred to a clinical psychologist or psychiatrist, according to the nature of their problem.

Those who remain depressed despite appropriate antidepressant medication in the right dosage for 4–6 months should be referred for psychiatric assessment to determine the factors which are maintaining the illness and whether other interventions are necessary, such as cognitive therapy.[17,18]

When anxiety persists despite anxiety management training from a clinical psychologist or the short-term use of benzodiazepines (for no longer than 2–4 weeks), a psychiatric opinion should be sought. Sexual problems usually respond to the Masters and Johnson approach.[19] Pre-existing marital problems which are worsened by the strain of the illness and its treatment can be difficult to resolve but merit intense intervention.

AFTER BEREAVEMENT

Despite considerable improvement in the outlook for children with cancer up to 50% will still die from it. There is, therefore, a need to consider how best to help parents who lose a child. Some centres attempt to follow-up every parent but it is clear that some parents wish to be left alone. Others welcome follow-up and the chance to talk through their feelings about what happened with a specialist nurse or social worker. Some centres hold support groups for bereaved parents.

REFERENCES

1. Maguire G. P. (1983), The psychological sequelae of childhood leukaemia in recent results in cancer research, in *Paediatric Oncology*, (Duncan W. R., ed.), Berlin, Springer Verlag, 47–56.
2. Tiller J. W. G., Ekert H., Rickards W. S. (1977), Family reactions in childhood acute lymphoblastic leukaemia in remission, *Austr. Paed. J.*; **13**: 178–81.
3. Marten, G. W., Goff J. R., Pownzek M., Payne J. S. (1979), *Psychosocial Evaluation of Children with Cancer: Care of the Child with Cancer* New York, American Cancer Society.
4. Magni G., Messina C., De Leo D., Mosconi A., Carli M. (1983), Psychological distress in parents of children with acute lymphatic leukaemia, *Acta Psychiatr. Scand.*; **68**; 297–300.
5. Peck B. (1979), Effects of childhood cancer on long term survivors and their families, *Br. Med. J.*; **1**: 1327–9.
6. Michelutte R., Patterson R. B., Herndon A. (1981), Evaluation of a home visitation programme for families of children with cancer, *Am. J. Ped. Haem. Oncol.*; **3**: 239–45.
7. Maguire P., Tait A., Brooke M., Thomas C., Sellwood R. (1980), Effect of counselling on the psychiatric morbidity associated with mastectomy, *Br. Med. J.*; **281**: 1454–6.
8. Watson M. (1983), Psychosocial intervention with cancer patients: a review, *Psychol. Med.*; **13**: 839–46.
9. Morrow G. R., Hoagland A. C., Morse I. P. (1982), Sources of support perceived by parents of children with cancer, *Patient Counsel. Hlth Ed.*; **4**: 36–40.
10. Adams M. A. (1978), Helping the parents of children with malignancy, *J. Pediat.*; **93**: 734–8.
11. Churven P. (1977), A group approach to the emotional needs of parents with leukaemic children, *Austr. Paed. J.*; **13**: 290–4.

12. Mantell J. E. (1983), Cancer patient visitor programmes: a case for account-ability, *J. Psychosoc. Oncol.*; 1: 45–58.
13. Steutzer C., Fuchtman D., Schulman J. L. (1976), Mothers as volunteers in an oncology clinic, *J. Ped.*; 5; 847–8.
14. Kaplan D. M., Grobstein R., Smith A. (1976), Predicting the impact of severe illness on families, *Health Soc. Work*; 1: 71–82.
15. Fife B. L. (1978), Reducing parental over protection of the leukaemic child, *Soc. Sci. Med.*; 12: 117–22.
16. Faulkner A., Maguire P. (1984), Training ward nurses to monitor cancer patients, *Clin. Oncol.*; 9: 319–24.
17. Goddard A. (1982), Cognitive behaviour therapy and depression, *Br. J. Hosp. Med.*; 27: 248–50.
18. Tarrier N., Maguire P., Kincey J. (1983), Locus of control and cognitive be-haviour therapy with mastectomy patients: a pilot study, *Br. J. Med. Psychol.*; 56: 265–70.
19. Masters M. H., Johnson V. E. (1970), *Human Sexual Inadequacy*, London, Churchill.

10

Helping women adapt to breast cancer

Peter Maguire and Ronald Sellwood

INTRODUCTION

When a woman presents to hospital with a breast lump that could be cancerous it is important to maximize her chances of adaptation by establishing her need for information and tailoring what is said accordingly.

First contact

When there is a definite possibility or probability that she has cancer of the breast it is important that she should be given a clear warning. Thus, the surgeon should say, for example: 'I have had a good look at you. This lump of yours could be harmless but it may not be so straightforward.' Once the surgeon has given a warning there must be a pause to allow the patient an opportunity to respond. It is possible that she would rather not know that her lump is cancerous and so she may respond: 'Oh, in that case I'll leave it all to you, you're the expert.' This is a clear signal that she does not want to know any more and the surgeon should accept this.

It is more likely that when she hears the phrase 'not so straightforward' she will respond: 'What do you mean, it's not so straightforward?' The surgeon should then give a further hint that it is serious by saying: 'Well, it could be a small tumour.' Providing that there is a further pause the patient will have a chance to indicate that she does not want to know anymore or ask 'What do you mean, a tumour?' The surgeon should then admit: 'Well, I think there could be some cancer there. We will need to have a look at your lump under a microscope to make sure.' Another pause will give an opportunity for this information to be digested and enable the woman to express her upset.

It is probable that she will be upset and it is important that this is acknowledged. This will indicate that it is legitimate for her to express her concerns overtly and make it likely that she will also be more honest about any problems that develop in the future. Thus, the surgeon should respond by saying: 'I can see you are upset, would you like to talk about it?' Most women will respond constructively by explaining why they are upset, for example, by saying: 'It's what I have been dreading.' The surgeon can then explore the reasons for this and may be faced with the following reply: 'My mother died from breast cancer. I have always dreaded that I would get it. She went very quickly, only 6 months after they found it. I have been terrified that I will get breast cancer myself and that I would die as quickly. How long have I got?'

When faced with such a reaction it is important that the surgeon should acknowledge that her fears are reasonable given her experience, but then try to maintain hope.

Surgeon: Given what happened to your mother I can understand why you have dreaded having cancer of the breast and why you are now worried that your lump could be cancer. Obviously, the only way I can confirm it is to do a biopsy and then tell you what I think is going on. However, from my examination and the tests we have run so far I do not think we are talking in terms of you lasting only 6 months. I think it's quite localized and you should be all right in the long term. But I will only be able to tell you this once we have the biopsy and some other tests. Is that OK?'

Patient: Yes.

Surgeon: I realize it is going to be very difficult for you until I can let you know what's happening, but I do believe that it's not going to turn out as badly as in your mother's case.

Patient: I hope so.

When the surgeon initially indicates that the lump could be more serious there may be no response from the patient to indicate whether she wants to know or prefers to leave it in the surgeons hands. When this happens the patient should be asked directly: 'Have you any questions? Are you sure?'

When the diagnosis is confirmed

Ideally the surgeon will try to separate diagnosis from treatment since this will give him time to discuss the diagnosis before considering treatment options. Otherwise the woman will tend to prefer to believe that the possibility of cancer is hypothetical and will not listen to any advice about possible treatments. It is important for the surgeon to fire a warning shot by indicating that the lump has turned out to be serious and needs further treatment.

Surgeon: From the needle biopsy that we did when you came to the clinic it has turned out to be more serious than I thought. From the x-rays we took it does seem to be a small cancer but I am hopeful that we will be able to remove it completely.

If the surgeon suspects that the cancer may be more serious a clear indication should be given without alarming the woman unduly, by saying, for example:

Surgeon: Well, as I warned you it has turned out to be cancerous. I would like to do some more x-rays just to check the state of play. How do you feel about that?'
Patient: Do you mean you are worried that it might have spread?
Surgeon: Yes, it is a possibility that some of the cells may have spread. So I think we ought to make sure.
Patient: And will you tell me if it has?
Surgeon: I'll certainly put you in the picture, but even if it has spread I am still hopeful that we can control it.

Here, the surgeon is not talking in terms of cure but of control. This will usually be sufficient to encourage the woman to believe that something can still be done.

As well as confirming the diagnosis the surgeon should mention the treatment that he would prefer to carry out. With an early cancer this could be a wide local excision plus a course of radiotherapy, or a mastectomy alone. It facilitates adaptation if the surgeon indicates a preference but allows the patient time to discuss this.

Surgeon: As it is small I would prefer just to remove the lump and then give you a course of radiotherapy.
Patient: Radiotherapy! Does that mean you are worried that not all the cancer cells will be taken away by surgery?
Surgeon: I am not particularly worried but it is a way of ensuring that any remaining cancer cells are destroyed by the radiotherapy.
Patient: I would rather have a mastectomy. That should make sure that all the cancer is removed. I have heard some terrible tales about radiotherapy. I would rather not have to go to the cancer hospital for it.
Surgeon: Well, we'd better sit down and look at the pros and cons of these two treatments then.

In discussing treatment options it is important to be honest about possible physical, social and psychological adverse effects so that the patient is sufficiently well informed that she can make a decision or discuss her situation with her partner. It is particularly important to avoid euphemisms like: 'The radiotherapy will make you a little sick' rather than: 'The radiotherapy can make some people feel very sick but if that happens you must tell us and we will do our best to reduce it.'

This frank discussion of options may greatly reduce the possibility of later psychological and social morbidity. If the surgeon feels there is insufficient time to explore options with the patient, a specialist nurse, social worker or patients who themselves have had breast cancer and surgery but have been selected and trained as volunteers may be used.

After surgery

After surgery the surgeon should be prepared to check how each woman has reacted to having a lumpectomy, wide local excision or mastectomy. Thus, the surgeon might ask: 'You know we had to remove your breast after all; how do you feel about that?' If the patient reacts by saying 'Terrible' it is then important that willingness to follow that up is shown by saying: 'What do you mean, terrible?' This gives the patient a chance to indicate if she is fearful of the cancer ('I keep thinking that it is going to spread to all parts of my body and kill me'), worried about losing a breast ('I'm so upset, I can't ever see myself feeling like a woman again'), or a combination of both ('I'm not sure which is worst, having cancer or losing a breast – I think they are both just as upsetting').

Assessment when the patient is still on the ward can be misleading and falsely optimistic. Many women feel cocooned and protected and do not think about the problems they may encounter on their return home. Even so, they need to be advised about exercises that could minimize swelling and pain in the arm affected by surgery, particularly if an axillary clearance was carried out to remove and check the lymph nodes. They should also be told about the prostheses available and encouraged to take the chosen prosthesis home for a trial period. This advice about exercises and prostheses can be provided by ward nurses, a specialist nurse, social worker, volunteer or through group meetings held on the ward.

Before the woman is discharged from hospital it is important that the surgeon should discuss any further investigations and treatments, e.g. whether or not to have radiotherapy or chemotherapy. When further treatments are indicated, it is important to be honest about why these are needed. Thus, when faced with a patient who needs chemotherapy because the lymph nodes were found to contain cancer cells the patient can be told, as follows:

Surgeon: As you know, the lump in your breast was small. But we found that when we removed some of the lymph nodes from under your arm some cancer cells had escaped there. Fortunately there is no evidence that they are anywhere else and your scan is clear. However, given that the nodes in your arm were involved I think we should give you some drugs which will mop up any remaining cancer cells.

Patient: Do you mean chemotherapy?

Surgeon: Well, yes, and they are strong drugs. They have to be in order to kill off the cancer cells. Because of that they can make you feel ill. They can make you feel very sick and put you off your food. But if there are any such side-effects you must tell us. We can then try to reduce them. On the other hand you may find that they do not affect you as badly as that. We'll need to give you them throughout the first year.

Similarly, with other treatments like radiotherapy it is important to indicate common adverse effects honestly rather than use euphemisms like: 'You'll only feel slightly tired.' It is probable that patients will feel much more tired than they were led to expect and this will cause them to distrust the surgeon.

After discharge

When patients attend follow-up clinics the surgeon should be prepared to check how they are adapting to the psychological hurdles posed by their disease.

Uncertainty

Any woman with breast cancer who knows her diagnosis has to come to terms with the terrible uncertainty that the cancer could come back at any time, causing suffering and a premature death. Some women are so plagued by this uncertainty that they cannot get thoughts of cancer out of their minds and their lives begin to be blighted by these worries. It is therefore important that their view of the future should be monitored by asking: 'How do you feel that your illness is going to work out?' This will allow the woman to indicate that she is very worried about her prognosis or that she is content to 'live a day at a time' and is able to forget that she has anything seriously wrong with her.

If the patient indicates that she has problems with uncertainty it is important to acknowledge and legitimize this:

Patient: I just can't stop thinking that the cancer could recur and kill me.
Surgeon: Well, you are right that it could eventually recur. This uncertainty
must be very difficult for you.
Patient: Yes, it's awful.
Surgeon: Well, the good news is that at the moment, as far as we can see from
your scan and physical examination, you are absolutely clear. How
often would you like me to see you to try and put your mind at rest?
Patient: Well, unless anything untoward happens, I think about every 3
months would help me keep going.
Surgeon: Well, I am prepared to see you on that basis but don't forget that
you must get in touch with me if you notice any signs that worry
you in between your 3-monthly visits.

By giving her regular markers of her progress and providing rapid access
the surgeon will help to reduce her uncertainty and improve her chances of
coping with the cancer.

Search for meaning

Unfortunately, medical science has still no adequate explanation to account
for why a given patient develops breast cancer ('Why me, why now?'). In the
absence of an adequate explanation patients search for other reasons. Two
theories are commonly implicated. Patients believe they developed cancer
because they were not able to cope with recent stress like a divorce or bereavement. Alternatively they may attribute cancer to their 'type C' personality. They have always bottled up their feelings, especially anger – 'It's bad
enough having cancer but to think it's your fault as well is the last straw.'[7]

Women may also look to sources outside themselves to explain the illness.
For example, they may blame their husband's cruelty, an apparent misdiag-
nosis of an earlier lump, or undue and unfair pressures at work. Since these
ideas usually hinder adaptation it is important to ask each patient whether
she has any explanation as to why she developed breast cancer. If such ideas
are evident it is important to explain that there is no objective evidence to
justify ideas that an inability to cope with internal or external stress or difficulties within one's personality cause cancer.

Control

With an illness like coronary heart disease (see Chapter 4) it is possible for
patients to feel hopeful because there are active steps they can take to reduce
the chance of a further heart attack. Thus, they may take up exercise and

change their diet. With breast cancer no such clear risk factors have been established. Consequently, some patients may feel that there is nothing they can do to combat their disease. This may provoke a feeling of helplessness, which may lead to a depressive illness. Some patients believe that selecting a special diet, taking up exercise or psychological activities like meditation will improve their chances of survival, so it is important to ask patients whether they feel that there is anything *they* can do to combat their illness. Those who express feelings of helplessness should be assessed for signs and symptoms of depression, as discussed below.

Stigma

Cancer is still perceived as the most feared disease in western society. People who develop cancer of the breast often feel singled out for misfortune and feel stigmatized. They feel that it will make them less attractive and acceptable to other people and they may use phrases like 'It's contagious' or 'leprosy' to describe this. Such feelings of stigma are not surprising given conventional views about possible causes of cancer. Women may have heard about theories that viruses may cause cancer or know that some cancers, like cancer of the cervix, are associated with promiscuity or venereal disease. Such theories increase worries that cancer can be passed from or to other people. Feelings of stigma may be so strong that they lead to social avoidance, sometimes leading to social isolation. The presence of stigma can be checked by asking: 'Has having cancer affected how you feel about yourself?' and 'Has it affected the amount of time you are seeing other people?' Where social withdrawal is evident the reasons for this should be explored and the patient should be encouraged to return to her premorbid level of social activity.

Openness

Women with breast cancer can find it very difficult to decide how open they should be with close relatives and friends about their illness and treatment. They worry that openness might jeopardize relationships and that people will not know how to respond to them because cancer and its treatments are not comfortable topics to talk about. Yet if the diagnosis is kept secret it will not be easy for the patient to make an adequate adaptation. It is helpful, therefore, to ask: 'Have you felt able to tell people close to you about your illness?' and then to add: 'What about other people?' If the patient has not been open it is important to explore the reasons why and then to encourage her to be open, at least with her partner. The patient may also raise the issue of openness with young children. Here it is useful to suggest that she should certainly give the children some warning that she has been ill but not discuss it in detail unless the child asks questions.

Reaction of other people

Because of fears of cancer, friends and relatives may find it difficult to know what to say to reassure the woman with cancer of the breast who is undergoing treatment. They may prefer to switch the conversation to neutral matters or to see less of the person than they did before her illness. There is then a risk that the patient will become isolated from the people who give her support. This will make her more vulnerable to psychological distress and psychiatric illness. It is important to ask each patient if she feels that her illness has in any way affected the behaviour of other people towards her. Sometimes the change will have been favourable in that the illness will have brought her much closer to key relatives and friends. But if isolation has occurred it is important to probe the nature and extent of this and to see whether anything practical can be done to re-establish contacts.

Medical support

Because it has to cope with so many patients the cancer centre may assume that the general practitioner will provide the patient with emotional support. However, patients generally perceive their practitioners as having insufficient up-to-date knowledge about breast cancer and so look to the hospital for information and support. Consequently, the patient may be given no help. Each patient should therefore be asked if she feels that her general practitioner and specialist have given her sufficient support and if she feels that they understood how she has reacted. Similarly, if the patient is being followed up by a specialist or community nurse it is worth checking whether she is finding this helpful or not and exploring the reasons for any dissatisfaction. This may well bring important but undisclosed problems to light.

TREATMENT-RELATED HURDLES

The patient should be asked how she has been affected by the treatment she has undergone or is still undergoing since it has been established that patients are reluctant to disclose any problems spontaneously. They perceive doctors and nurses who are involved in their care as being busy. They do not want to burden them further and fear that the treatment of their cancer might be neglected if they volunteer emotional problems. They also worry that they will be seen as inadequate and ungrateful because they are the only patients who are not coping. The belief that the problems they are experiencing are inevitable and that nothing can be done to alleviate them is common. Thus it is essential to ask each woman how she felt about her surgery and clarify her responses:

Surgeon: How have you felt about losing a breast?
Patient: Devastated, absolutely devastated.
Surgeon: In what way, devastated?
Patient: I feel so repulsive. I can't bear to look at myself – I feel a freak – I can't let my husband near me.
Surgeon: Is that causing problems with your husband?
Patient: He insists that he does not mind – but I find it hard to believe him.

It is also important to elicit the impact of surgery even when it has been possible to conserve the breast.

Surgeon: How have you felt about your surgery?
Patient: Not so good. I keep worrying that some cancer cells must have been left behind and are still there despite the radiotherapy. My other breast is larger and I'm beginning to feel lop-sided. It is making me quite self-conscious.

In exploring possible body image problems it is important to remember that there are three categories which can occur separately or in combination. The patient may be concerned that she is no longer physically whole and feels vulnerable psychologically. She may have developed a heightened self-consciousness and worry that other people must realize that she has lost a breast even if she wears baggy clothes to conceal her shape. She may feel that the loss of a breast has made her feel less feminine and attractive. If such body image problems are present it is important to determine how much she avoids looking at her chest wall when dressing, undressing or bathing. If she avoids looking, her reasons for this should be explored.

Surgeon: Why do you avoid looking?
Patient: I hate how I look – I feel ugly – how can anyone like me again?
Surgeon: Any other reasons why you cannot look?
Patient: It reminds me that I have had cancer.

About 1 in 10 women develop persistent swelling and pain in the arm when an axillary clearance is carried out. This can be debilitating and frustrate the woman's attempts to return to work. The extent to which her arm has recovered should be explored and the nature and extent of any pain or swelling established.

If the patient is undergoing radiotherapy it is important to establish her perceptions of it and its impact.

Surgeon: How are you feeling about having radiotherapy?
Patient: I have been very worried.
Surgeon: What have you been worried about?
Patient: I keep thinking you must have left some cancer cells behind. Otherwise, I wouldn't need radiotherapy.
Surgeon: How's the radiotherapy affecting you?
Patient: It is making me feel very tired.

When tiredness is persisting the possibility of the patient having developed a depressive illness should be explored (see below).

When adjuvant chemotherapy is used it often causes adverse effects, particularly on the gastrointestinal tract. It may also result in the development of conditioned responses. Here any mention, sound or smell which reminds the patient of chemotherapy can then lead her to feel nauseous or to vomit. If this conditioning is not treated she may become too fearful of treatment and opt out. Otherwise, she will feel in a terrible dilemma. Her life depends on the treatment but she is finding it increasingly difficult to continue. There is a strong link between such adverse effects and conditioning and the later development of an anxiety state, depressive illness or both.

Both radiotherapy and chemotherapy can affect sexual functioning adversely. If radiotherapy is used to oblate the ovaries in a premenopausal woman it will lead to an artificial menopause, infertility and loss of libido. Chemotherapy can also cause a premature menopause, infertility and loss of libido because it reduces oestrogen levels, and increases follicular stimulating and luteinizing hormones. It is helpful therefore to ask any women on radiotherapy or chemotherapy if it has had any effect on her personal relationships, particularly her sexual functioning. Otherwise there is a strong risk that she will not disclose such a personal problem.

GENERAL ADJUSTMENT

It is important to check whether the woman has yet returned to work, taken up her previous social and leisure activities and is coping with her household chores as well as she was before surgery.

WHO SHOULD ASSESS?

Ideally, the surgeon or general practitioner will find time to ask the relevant questions during routine outpatient visits or visits to the surgery. However, surgeons or practitioners may worry that such enquiries will take up too much of their time and fear that they could be faced with difficulties which they are not confident that they can handle. For example, they might be asked difficult questions about prognosis or treatment options. They also worry that they may be faced with strong emotions like anger or despair which they do not have the time or expertise to deal with adequately. There is then a danger that they will use distancing tactics to avoid a dialogue developing. If they use such tactics the chances of problems being disclosed will be minimal. These distancing strategies include premature reassurance.

Surgeon: I think we should bring you in to have a look at that lump under a
microscope.
Patient: Does that mean it's serious?
Surgeon: Well, it could be. I can see you are upset but there is no need to be,
we'll get you in in no time. I am sure that it is going to be all right.

Here, the surgeon has allowed the patient no opportunity to explain why she was upset. So, his reassurance may have been misdirected and inappropriate. Other commonly used distancing tactics include preferential attention to physical rather than psychological matters and premature problem-solving, as when the moment a doctor hears a problem he tries to solve it rather than exploring whether there were any other problems before deciding on the best management strategy. Because of these distancing tactics and the lack of adequate training in interviewing, assessment and counselling skills, the surgeon or practitioner may feel ill equipped to carry out the psychological assessment. Alternatively, he may genuinely believe that he has not sufficient time to do it. He should then consider nominating a member of his team to do this monitoring or employ a specialist nurse to help.

ROLE OF SPECIALIST NURSES

Full intervention

In one study specialist nurses were trained to provide counselling before and after mastectomy and then to monitor progress by asking questions, such as those already discussed above. They assessed each woman every 2 months after discharge for the first year. They were able to recognize most of the patients who developed physical, psychological or sexual problems, whereas few problems were recognized in a control group who were not followed up in the same way.[1] However, this intensive follow-up created difficulties. Both ward and clinic nurses felt that their jobs were being threatened. Women with breast cancer tended to look to the specialist nurses to help them with problems unrelated to mastectomy. The nurses were faced with a steadily accumulating load of patients. They found it especially difficult when patients they had come to know well developed a recurrence of cancer and died. The nurses also found that some of the women they visited did not find counselling helpful and would have preferred to have been left alone. Consequently, an alternative approach was tried, that of limited intervention.

Limited intervention

The specialist nurses were asked to limit their involvement to pre- and postoperative counselling and one home visit within a month of discharge, when a full assessment was carried out. Thereafter, the onus was put on patients to contact the nurse if any problems arose. It was hoped this would minimize patients' dependence on the nurse, allowing her to concentrate on those patients who most needed help. It proved to be as effective as the full intervention scheme and a practical cost-effective way of monitoring women with breast cancer. It ensured as far as possible their rapid restoration to a reasonable level of functioning through the early recognition and treatment of any problems.

USE OF OTHER NURSES

The employment of specialist nurses can lead other nurses and doctors to rely on them to carry out the necessary monitoring and rehabilitation, and they then become less skilled on delivering this care. The specialist nurses are expected to take on all patients with breast cancer. Therefore, it is useful to consider whether non-specialist nurses working on a surgical ward or in the community could monitor the progress of women with breast cancer. Hence, ward nurses and community nurses were trained in the same counselling and assessment skills as the specialist nurses to determine if they would prove as effective. While the ward nurses showed a significant improvement in their ability to recognize which patients developed problems while on the ward,[2] the nurses working in the community failed to improve. Indeed, some actually deteriorated in their ability to assess the progress of women with breast cancer. There were several reasons. They felt that they were already overburdened with looking after patients. They were not confident that they would be given appropriate back-up if they found that women had psychological and social problems which needed intervention. They did not believe they had adequate support from their nurse managers or general practitioners. They thought it preferable to continue to use distancing strategies in order to avoid real dialogue with women with breast cancer about any problems due to their disease or treatment.

Suggested solutions

A consensus meeting held by the King Edward's Fund concluded that the best solution would be to employ a specialist nurse within each health district to help rehabilitate women with breast cancer. It was emphasized that such nurses need adequate support from surgeons, general practitioners, clinical psychologists and psychiatrists if the problems they uncover are to be treated adequately. Such a nurse would work most effectively if ward nurses were trained to provide basic information, advice and emotional support while the patient is in hospital. This would free the specialist nurse to concentrate on those who had already developed problems or who needed particular help. After discharge, those health visitors and district nurses who were interested could be enlisted to monitor patients and so free the specialist nurse to concentrate on those most at risk. The specialist nurse would refer patients with problems in the first instance to the general practitioner. If the general practitioner felt more expert help was needed the specialist nurse would have direct and prompt access to a clinical psychologist and/or psychiatrist.

INTERVENTION

Depressive illness

At least 1 in 4 women with breast cancer will develop a depressive illness after mastectomy.[3,4] The woman will report that she has been feeling persistently low and miserable to an extent which represents a distinct difference from her normal self. She cannot distract herself out of this low mood or be distracted by others. She will also complain of at least four other symptoms of depression [irritability, impairment of concentration, forgetfulness, loss or increase in weight, loss of libido, loss of energy, fatiguability, sleep disturbance (repeated waking or early-morning waking), feelings of hopelessness, guilt, worthlessness, feeling a burden, experiencing suicidal ideas, agitation or retardation]. It is important to realize that depression is an illness and to avoid dismissing it as an understandable reaction which does not merit attention. If the depression has persisted for 4 weeks or more or is severe, it should be treated promptly with an appropriate antidepressant. It is essential to choose an antidepressant which will cause the fewest side-effects. This will prevent the patient wrongly attributing any side-effects to recurrence or spread and will improve compliance. The rationale for treating her depression should be explained to the patient on the basis that the strain of the illness or surgery has provoked an illness which, though understandable, requires a drug to correct the biochemical change. It must be emphasized that the drug is not a tranquillizer and to warn her that there could be side-effects like dry mouth or drowsiness. The chosen antidepressant should be given in effective dosage and continued for 4–6 months to prevent relapse.

Anxiety state

An anxiety state should be considered when the woman complains that she is plagued by worry and is unable to stop worrying about the cancer or surgery. She also complains of being unable to relax and of feeling constantly on edge and tense. There will also be other symptoms of anxiety, including difficulty getting off to sleep, irritability, poor concentration and indecisiveness. Physical symptoms like palpitations, sweating, headache, breathlessness, shakiness and tremor are likely to be prominent.

Sometimes anxiety presents as an agoraphobic state where the woman is afraid of going out of the house alone in case she collapses. There is usually then a pattern of avoiding crowds and busy shops, particularly supermarkets, and travelling on buses.

Occasionally, a woman will present with a cancer phobia. Though she is free of disease and has been told so she remains terrified that she has cancer in the remaining breast or has developed a recurrence. She may have also developed a habit of examining her breast repeatedly to check for further cancer and may have begun to seek reassurance frequently from her general practitioner or surgeon. If the anxiety is overwhelming and the patient's ability to function is impaired, an anxiolytic, such as a benzodiazepine, should be used in the short term, that is up to 2–3 weeks. When somatic aspects predominate a beta-blocker, such as propanolol, may be tried. If the woman is agitated and disorganized a major tranquillizer, such as thioridazine or chlorpromazine, should be considered.

Many patients suffering from anxiety benefit from being taught progressive muscular relacation.[5] Instructional audiotapes can assist this. The patients are then asked to employ these relaxation techniques whenever they feel anxious or are about to confront anxiety-provoking situations. Patients can also be taught to summon up tranquil scenes to distract themselves and banish unwanted and upsetting thoughts.

Desensitization is a useful treatment if the patient has developed agoraphobia, social or cancer phobia. The therapist first constructs a hierarchy of situations or thoughts which are most or least likely to provoke anxiety. The woman is then taught to relax and asked to imagine an item low on the hierarchy, for example: 'I worry about cancer when my breast feels sore'. If she can imagine this without becoming anxious she moves on to the next item in the hierarchy. When the woman has agoraphobia she is asked to imagine confronting situations while trying to relax and then to confront them in real life. Such graded exposure is often effective. Women with cancer phobia who examine themselves repeatedly can also benefit from being taught anxiety management techniques as well as distraction and thought-stopping.

Body image problems

The use of progressive muscular relaxation and desensitization to help a woman look at her chest wall, first in imagination and then in real life, can also be effective. However, in some women the body image problems remain and a more cognitive approach is required. This involves challenging her assumptions that she is no longer attractive or of any use. Some women may reject psychological help and consider that only breast reconstruction will help. Women who want a reconstruction for themselves rather than because they are being pressed to have one by somebody else, are aware they will get a cleavage rather than a breast like the original, and who are realistic about the complications of plastic surgery respond well. Women who dislike the external prosthesis intensely because it slips around or reminds them of their cancer also benefit from reconstruction.

Conditioned responses

It is important to act promptly when the patient develops conditioning, or else she may opt out of treatment. Covering each major injection or infusion with an anxiolytic drug, such as lorazepam, a major tranquillizer, such as chorpromazine, and/or an anti-emetic may be sufficient. Teaching anxiety management techniques can also be effective.[6] It is also important to treat any associated depressive illness, as discussed previously.

Sexual problems

Most women respond well to the Masters and Johnson conjoint approach where the woman and her partner are helped together.[7] This begins with a ban on sexual intercourse in order to lessen the woman's fear of it. The couple are then encouraged to find ways of pleasuring each other which do not involve genital contact. Once they become confident in each other again they proceed towards full intercourse. A major barrier to this treatment can be the woman's inability to accept her breast loss. She will then need desensitization or breast reconstruction before therapy can proceed. The sexual problem may often be overcome by reconstruction alone.

USE OF VOLUNTEERS AND SELF-HELP GROUPS

During the period of diagnosis and treatment the patient may wish to talk to other women who have had similar experiences and who wish to help others. As yet, there have been no adequate control studies of the effect of such volunteers, but anecdotally, some patients have found them helpful. It is important that they should be chosen carefully.[8] They should be able to listen, be sensible in their approach, avoid imposing their own experiences on the patient, and help her to explore her own options rather than advising solutions. Otherwise it is possible they may cause more psychological harm than good.

Many districts have established self-help groups. These can be effective provided they are controlled by leaders who have a knowledge of group dynamics and can help the group work constructively by encouraging women to discuss real problems, rather than becoming a psychotherapy group where inappropriate levels of personal disclosure are allowed. Properly conducted groups can help women to feel less isolated after mastectomy or other treatments and to gain support from each other. They can also provide practical advice and information. Unfortunately, only 1 in 10 of women with breast cancer are likely to use such support groups consistently.

CONCLUSIONS

The rehabilitation of women who undergo treatment for breast cancer would be much advanced by the appointment of specialist nurses within each health district; these nurses would work closely with the surgeon, general practitioner and back-up psychologist and psychiatrist to ensure that any problems which are not prevented by counselling are recognized rapidly and treated.

REFERENCES

1. Maguire P., Tait A., Brooke M., Thomas C., Sellwood R. (1980), Effect of counselling on the psychiatric morbidity associated with mastectomy, *Br. Med. J.*; **281**: 1454–6.
2. Faulkner A., Maguire P. (1984), Teaching ward nurses to monitor cancer patients, *Clin. Oncol.*; **10**: 383–9.
3. Morris T. (1979), Psychological adjustment to mastectomy, *Cancer Treat. Rev.*; **6**: 41–61.
4. Maguire G. P., Lee E. G., Bevington D. J. et al (1978), Psychiatric problems in the first year after mastectomy, *Br. Med. J.*; **1**: 963–5.
5. Janoun L., Oppenheimer C., Gelder M. (1962), A self-help treatment programme for anxiety-state patients, *Behaviour Therapy*; **13**: 103–11.
6. Morrow G. R., Morrell C. (1982), The antiemetic efficacy of behavioural treatment for cancer chemotherapy-induced anticipatory nausea and vomiting, *N. Engl. J. Med.*; **307**: 1476–80.
7. Masters M. H., Johnson V. E. (1980), *Human sexual inadequacy*, 2nd edn, London, Bantam Books.
8. Mantell J. E. (1983), Cancer patient visitor programmes: a case for accountability, *J. Psychosoc. Oncol.*; **1**: 45–53.

11

Rehabilitation of patients with a stoma

Nan Brady and Peter Maguire

INTRODUCTION

The formation of a stoma inevitably alters the patient's body image and this can have far-reaching psychological implications, since the mental picture each person has of his or her own body encompasses physical appearance, physical activities, personal relationships and social life. Surgery challenges this picture and forces a reappraisal. While some patients can develop and assimilate a new picture and still retain their personal identity and feelings of worth, others fail to do so and suffer psychological morbidity.

PSYCHOLOGICAL MORBIDITY

Body image problems

Patients have to try to adapt both to the stoma and the colostomy bag. Some find the stoma hard to accept because it is a part of their bowel and should not be visible to the outside world. They may use phrases like 'obscene' and 'repulsive' to describe their responses to it. Others are more concerned about the workings of the bag. Despite the advent of good stoma bags patients may still fear that the bag will be visible to others, may smell, make noises, leak or burst. Body image problems may be intensified if patients know that they had a cancer removed. They may fear they are vulnerable to recurrence and feel stigmatized by having a socially unacceptable disease.

These body image problems become manifest in three ways. Up to one-third of patients feel very self-conscious about the stoma and ashamed and embarrassed.[1] This can result in a marked curtailment of their social and leisure activities which is maintained unless help is offered. At least 1 in 4 patients feel much less attractive and less masculine or feminine, whichever is applicable.

One-half of all stoma patients experience some feelings of stigma which can be severe and persistent in up to 20.[1] Younger patients seem most likely to feel stigmatized. As many as 23% think constantly about it because they believe that there is a constant risk that their stoma could become manifest to others through an 'accident'.

The formation of a stoma can also lead to a marked loss of self-esteem; patients so affected feel more vulnerable psychologically and physically to any subsequent adversity.

Affective disorders

Regardless of the disease which necessitated a stoma, between 20 and 25% of patients will develop an anxiety state and/or depressive illness within the first few years of surgery.[2][5] While most episodes are of only moderate severity some patients become severely depressed and may commit suicide. Few of these affective disorders appear to improve without help. Body image problems and feelings of stigma contribute strongly to the development of psychiatric problems.[1]

Occasionally, the affective disorder presents as a phobia of the stoma or bag. The patient cannot bear to look at the stoma or deal with the bag, relying on his or her partner to change it. Attempts to make patients look at their bags cause them to experience strong feelings of panic and to become disorganized.

Sexual problems

Between one-quarter to three-quarters of men with stomas complain of difficulty in obtaining and maintaining an erection or of problems with ejaculation.[6] Up to one-third of women experience a marked loss of sexual interest or enjoyment.[6] Some of these sexual problems are caused by surgical destruction of the nerves serving the genital organs. In other patients they are due to anxiety and depression.

Social morbidity

In addition to the marked reduction in the social and leisure activities of one-fifth of stoma patients, some patients fail to return to their previous level of working or housework even though they are physically fit to do so.[7]

Implications for rehabilitation

The aim of rehabilitation is to maximize the quality of life of stoma patients by helping restore them physically, socially and psychologically to as normal a life as possible, at the pace most suited to the individual. The challenge is how best to reduce the considerable physical, social and psychological morbidity. Given the link between failure to adapt and inadequate preparation, rehabilitation should begin before surgery.

REHABILITATION

Before surgery

When the surgery is elective the patient should be told that a stoma is necessary and given an opportunity to discuss the implications.

When emergency surgery is required, whenever possible the patient should be forewarned. He or she then has time to prepare psychologically for a stoma but may then be fortunate to learn that it was unnecessary. Otherwise, the news that he or she has had a stoma formed may come as a sudden shock and be hard to assimilate or promote denial.

A key issue is who should handle the discussions before surgery. Should it be the ward nurses or a clinical nurse specialist who is educated and trained in the knowledge and skills of stoma care? The preferred solution is to employ a specialist nurse. As a result of her training she will be best able to deal with the varying and complex needs of stoma patients. She can avoid fragmentation of care by taking a holistic approach – dealing with physical, social and psychological aspects – and liaising with all members of the hospital and community care team. By offering direct access to patients who require support and advice, she can hope to assess, help or refer most of those who develop problems after surgery.

At her initial contact preoperatively she can begin to assess and identify the problems and needs of each patient. She can then set reasonable objectives, negotiate these with the patient, decide how these will be achieved and monitor outcome.

The aim of this preoperative preparation is to explore how the patient and partner feel about the diagnosis, the intended surgery, the changes in body functioning and body image. The nurse also seeks to establish their needs for information and to respond appropriately. Thus, she will not move into an automatic sequence of advice, such as 'Let me tell you about your stoma'. . . . Instead, she will first check how much patients would like to know: 'Would you like to know more about this stoma? What exactly would you like to know?' She will then respond to each issue so raised: 'First let's look at your question about where it will be sited, then we'll talk about your worries about leakage and smell'.

It is important to ensure that *all* the patient's concerns have been identified before offering advice. Otherwise the advice will not be heeded because the patient is still preoccupied with those other concerns. Questions should be answered simply and honestly but an appropriate level of hope should be maintained, as in the following example.

Stoma nurse: Have you any other concerns?
Patient: Yes, isn't it going to smell?
Stoma nurse: There is a chance it could do, but I'm here to try to make sure it doesn't. If there are any problems with smell we should be able to do something about them.

Premature or false reassurance, as in the following example, should be avoided if a relationship of trust is to be established and maintained.

Patient: I am worried that it is going to smell.
Stoma nurse: There's absolutely no need to worry about that. We have such good bags these days. There will be no problems with smell.

The nurse's advice was premature because she did not explore the basis of her patient's worries. Had she done so she would have found out that the patient was fastidious about hygiene and physical appearance and profoundly upset at the prospect of smelling.

Insisting that there would be no problems with smell represented false reassurance and could promote serious distrust in the longer term.

From the outset the stoma nurse should educate the patient about his or her responsibility to learn to manage the stoma and maintain a good level of health, but that the nurse will be willing to help achieve these goals in the optimal time and will be available if any problems are encountered.

The site for placement of the stoma should be selected with the full participation of the patient and in the light of knowledge of lifestyle, occupation, culture, religion, clothes preference, leisure activities and physical disabilities. The importance of choosing the correct site cannot be over-emphasized. It leads to better control of the stoma and reduces the risks of leakage, odour, sore skin, loss of confidence and depression. Involving patients in the choice of site encourages them to take responsibility for their stomas.

If the patient wishes to talk to an ostomy visitor, a volunteer from the relevant association can be introduced now or this can be left until later. Meeting and speaking with a suitable volunteer allows the patient to see that it is possible to adapt to life with a stoma, whatever the initial problems.

After surgery

The patient is given a further opportunity to discuss any concerns about the illness. Those who have suffered from inflammatory bowel disease are likely to feel relieved that the days of pain, diarrhoea and frequent visits to the lavatory are now over. They may even see the stoma as bringing a new lease of life. In patients with long-term neurological disorders, such as multiple sclerosis, the creation of a stoma relieves urinary incontinence or constipation. This can do much to restore confidence and encourage them to tolerate their illness better. Patients who are aware they have had cancer removed will usually feel grateful, but may worry about recurrence. Fears of recurrence can then be triggered every time they look at the stoma.

Questions about longer-term survival such as: 'How long have I got?' are best dealt with by first checking why the patient is asking, since this will reveal what he or she is really asking. The answers should then be appropriate to the patient's prognosis.

Patient: How long have I got?

Stoma nurse: I'd be happy to try to answer that but first it would help me if I knew why you were asking?

Patient: I know I had a cancer removed and I am worrying whether they got it all.

Stoma nurse: Any other reasons?

Patient: No.

Stoma nurse: Well, I gather they are pretty confident that they did get it all and that you should be OK.

Patient: But for how long?

Stoma nurse: That we can never tell for certain, and so I can't give you an answer. But we will be following you up to check how you are and even if we find anything we should still be able to do something.

Once concerns about illness have been dealt with the patient is taught how to care for the stoma and surrounding skin. Help is then given in assisting in the selection of the most suitable bag and other necessary equipment. Specific concerns about the stoma and bag should be explored and appropriate advice and reassurance offered. The stoma nurse should be especially alert to signs of an adverse reaction and willing to acknowledge these.

Stoma nurse: I get the feeling that you are not very happy about managing your bag.

Patient: You're right. I don't like it, not one bit.

Stoma nurse: Why not?
Patient: Its not natural, is it? I'm terrified I'll have an accident with it.

Industry, in co-operation with patients and professionals, has made excellent appliances and accessories available, which are obtained free of charge on prescription. Details of all essential equipment are given by the stoma care nurse to each patient and a copy of the information is sent to the general practitioner.

The patient and family are given instructions on how to obtain and store supplies and how to dispose of used equipment. The patient is also given a booklet containing helpful advice on diet, clothing, skin care, clinic times, addresses and telephone numbers of self-help groups and how to contact the stoma care nurse.

Monitoring progress

The progress of patients is monitored to check how they are adapting physically, socially and psychologically. Particular attention is paid to the patients' adaptation to the stoma and colostomy; 'How are you feeling about your stoma/colostomy? Have you been experiencing any difficulties?' The exact nature and extent of any problem can then be clarified. The stoma care nurse also checks the extent of the patients' social recovery; 'Are you back at work yet? Have you started going to bingo again?' and establishes the reasons for any delay. The impact of the stoma on key relationships and sexual functioning is also enquired about: 'Has having a stoma affected your relationship with your partner? In what way? Has the physical side of your relationship been affected in any way?' Finally, screening questions are asked to elicit any anxiety or depression: 'Have you, at any stage since your surgery, felt particularly worried, tense or unable to relax/felt especially low or miserable?' If mood disturbance is likely, follow-up questions are asked to check if other key signs and symptoms of anxiety and depression are present.

Resolving problems

The stoma nurse will seek to refer patients with body image problems to a clinical psychologist or psychiatrist for behaviour therapy, including relaxation training and desensitization to the stoma and bag through graded exposure. Patients with an anxiety state may also respond to anxiety management techniques taught by a clinical psychologist. Those with a depressive illness usually benefit from antidepressant therapy. This can be initiated by the general practitioner, surgical team or psychiatrist. When sexual problems are not due to surgical damage the Masters and Johnson method of conjoint sexual therapy can be effective. Otherwise, alternative ways of pleasuring may need to be suggested.

When such problems are evident it is important that the stoma care nurse should give feedback to the surgeon and general practitioner. This increases their awareness of the need for a rehabilitation programme and for active intervention when problems arise.

Those at risk

Children and adolescents

Some babies are born with defects to their bladder, bowel or anus and have a permanent or temporary stoma. News of this surgery can be shattering to patients. Their beautiful baby will be disfigured permanently. Great sensitivity is called for in reinforcing why such surgery is necessary and trying to minimize feelings of guilt and blame. Fortunately most stomas which are created in babies are temporary in nature but some are permanent. Going to school for the first time then represents a major challenge, since other children can be intolerant and unkind. It can be difficult to empty the bag with any degree of privacy but the provision of special arrangements may cause derision. Liaison with teachers, parents and the school nurse can assist in making the best use of available resources.

Patients who are going through puberty and adolescence and are trying to sort out their personal identity may find a stoma especially hard to cope with. Moreover, physical appearance and clothing are extremely important, as are encounters with the opposite sex. Fears of insecurity and rejection can be profound and intensive counselling may be needed to counteract those and promote emotional growth and self-esteem.

Others

Stoma patients with a previous psychiatric illness, who feel they had insufficient advice and information before and after surgery, and those who experience feelings of stigma and physical complications appear especially at risk of morbidity and warrant careful monitoring.[9]

Patients who predict that their partners will not be supportive merit special attention. It is important to verify whether these predictions are justified and to involve the partner in any case.

The anus is an erotic zone for some in our society and its absence can cause profound difficulties for homosexuals. The stoma care nurse must examine her own feelings and have respect for those of others in order to provide an understanding atmosphere in which the patient can fully express his feelings and concerns.

Patients who have no established partner may despair that they will ever find one. They need advice about how and when to disclose their stoma to a potential partner.

Older patients may find it difficult to adapt because of failing sight or arthritis. This can provide deep feelings of isolation and despondency. Great tact and patience are needed if such patients are to accept the offered help, which must respect their right to independence and privacy.

CONCLUSIONS

If rehabilitation is to be successful it must allow for variation in individual responses. While some patients may view the formation of a stoma as a life-saving procedure, others may find it an intolerable intrusion into their life-style. Rehabilitation must also help the patient find solutions rather than impose them through stereotyped advice and reassurance.

REFERENCES

1. MacDonald L. D., Anderson H. R. (1984), Stigma in patients with rectal cancer: a community study, *Epidemiol. Commun. Hlth*; **38**: 284–90.
2. Devlin H. B., Plant J. A., Griffin M. (1971), The aftermath of surgery for ano-rectal cancer, *Br. Med. J.*; **3**: 413–18.
3. Wirsching M., Druner H. V., Herman G. (1975), Results of psychological adjust-ment to long term colostomy, *Psychother. Psychosom.*; **26**: 245–56.
4. Thomas C., Madden F., Jehn D. (1987), Psychological effects of stomas. 1. Psychosocial morbidity 1 year after surgery, *J. Psychosom. Res.*; **31**: 311–16.
5. Williams N. S., Johnston D. (1983), The quality of life after rectal excision for low rectal cancer, *Br. J. Surgery*; **70**: 460–4.
6. Anderson B. L. (1985), Sexual functioning morbidity among cancer survivors, *Cancer*; **55**: 1835–42.
7. Eardley A., George W. D., Davis E. et al (1976), Colostomy: the consequence of surgery, *Clin. Oncol.*; **2**: 277–83.
8. Masters M. H., Johnson V. E. (1970), *Human Sexual Inadequacy*, London, Churchill.
9. Thomas C., Madden F., Jehn D. (1987), Psychological effects of stomas. II. Factors influencing outcome, *J. Psychosom. Res.*; **31**: 317–23.

12

The role of self-help groups in overcoming disability

A case study of the Spinal Injuries Association

Mike Oliver and Frances Hasler

INTRODUCTION

Throughout this book, the importance of the voluntary sector has been emphasized. Not only do charities create funds for research (such as the Arthritis and Rheumatism Council, the Chest, Heart and Stroke Association etc.) but also they may provide solely or in addition, services and facilities for people suffering from various conditions (Arthritis Care, the Multiple Sclerosis Society etc.).

Perhaps the most important function a self-help group can perform, however, is that of mutual support. Few professionals suffer from the disabilities which afflict their patients (clients). The intellectual grasp of what someone is feeling will always be different from the actual knowledge of what it is like when it happens to oneself. The Spinal Injuries Association has a major objective of helping individuals to achieve their own goals and all its full members are themselves spinally injured. It is appropriate, therefore, to examine in some detail its development and *modus operandi*.

The onset of disability in general and of spinal cord injury in particular may have profound implications for the person concerned and indeed for those who are close to him or her. Such onset is likely to be traumatic in origin and sudden in impact, necessitating immediate and acute medical intervention, firstly to save the injured person's life and then to stabilize his or her physical condition. Nursing intervention is also important to ensure that complications like pressure sores are not allowed to develop and as time passes physiotherapists and occupational therapists will become closely involved in the rehabilitation of the patient. Finally, social work intervention may also be necessary in order to facilitate the return of the spinal cord injured person to the community.

The above is a brief description of the process by which the spinal injured person is returned to the community following a traumatic accident. While it must be conceded that great progress has been made in the treatment, care and rehabilitation of people with spinal cord injury since the end of World War II, there are nonetheless a number of criticisms that can be levelled at the whole process. To begin with, medical and associated professions may be very good at dealing with the physical problems associated with spinal cord injury but are less skilled in dealing with other difficulties. In addition, helping the whole family rather than just the disabled individual is only just being recognized as an essential part of the process. Finally, return to the community is often met with delays in the supply of aids and equipment, lack of suitable housing and poor liaison and communication between the professionals concerned.

When the spinal injured person is returned to the community he or she will be faced with a range of difficulties concerning employment, finance, housing and the pursuit of leisure and social activities. Thus the range of difficulties likely to be faced can be divided into three discrete areas: physical, emotional and practical. Physical refers to the developing of the remaining bodily functions to their maximum and the restoration of physical health. Emotional difficulties are the adjustments that may need to be made in personal and social relationships consequent upon living life in a wheelchair. Practical problems are found when adopting a chosen lifestyle given that society is not organized to take into account the needs of people in wheelchairs.

The traditional medically dominated spinal injury service can not resolve these difficulties and there are aspects of physical care that can only be learned through the direct experience of spinal cord injury. As one person said: 'All the important things I learned about self-care, I learned from other paraplegics, not the professionals'. In the area of emotional difficulties, the general issues involved are not understood, let alone an appropriate service provided. (For a critique of existing theories of psychological adjustment to spinal cord injury, see Oliver.[1]) This has led Trieschmann in her review[2] to conclude that many people with spinal cord injury 'have felt victimized by professionals who write articles about the reactions to spinal cord injury which are based more on theory than fact.'

Finally, in the area of practical difficulties, the traditional service has not seen as its role the articulation of the practical problems faced by paraplegics living in society, and hence has not recognized a duty to act as an advocate in the political process necessary to bring about the necessary changes.

Thus the Spinal Injuries Association (SIA) was set up as a self-help group to begin to tackle some of these areas of difficulty. It was not established, however, in opposition to the spinal injury service but rather as a complement to it, as the limits of medicine and the medically dominated services were being recognized even by some members of the medical profession. However the establishment of the SIA was not merely a response to some of the issues discussed above but part of a wider social movement which saw the mushrooming and development of many self-help groups in the late 1960s and early 1970s. Before going on to discuss in detail the SIA, we need therefore to locate the rise of self-help groups in an appropriate context.

SELF-HELP IN A HISTORICAL CONTEXT

The origins of the self-help movement arose in the nineteenth rather than the twentieth century as a response to the industrialization process in Britain. As far as self-help was concerned, there were two aspects – individual and collective. Individual self-help was a requirement of the majority of individual wage labourers who made up the mass of workers in the new factory system and this was epitomized by Samuel Smiles.[3] The collective self-help response was largely through the creation of working men's organizations, notably Friendly Societies and Voluntary Provident Associations. 'In essence many of them owed their origins to the need felt by working men to provide themselves with succour against the poverty and destitution resulting from sickness and death at a time when the community offered only resort to the overseer of the poor'.[4]

However, by the early twentieth century the conditions which had given rise to such self-help responses were changing. Old age pensions were being introduced, the working week was gradually shortened, more and more workers were entitled to annual holidays and there were widening opportunities for recreation and social activities. The founding of the Welfare State after World War II further weakened the need for self-help. However, immediate post-war optimism had within twenty years given way to disillusion and a gradual realization that the Welfare State could not meet the needs of all the people all of the time. It could not in fact, as its originators had hoped, provide 'cradle-to-grave' security.

So the 1960s and early 1970s saw a rebirth of self-help as a response to the changed social conditions of the late twentieth century. Firstly, there was disillusion over the professionalization of much of what had been done by individuals for themselves or for each other. Secondly, supportive social institutions like the family and the neighbourhood community were undergoing changes and coming under the increasing pressures of urbanization. Thirdly, the complexity and size of new institutions and communities left people feeling depersonalized and dehumanized. Finally, and specifically in relation to health, there was the failure of medicine to provide universal cures and the subsequent inability of the NHS to provide appropriate care for those who could not be cured. This last factor was an important element in the formation and development of the SIA, for there is no cure for spinal cord injury and, as has already been pointed out, a number of criticisms could be levelled at the traditional model of caring for people with spinal cord injury.

Robinson and Henry[5] in their important study of self-help in the area of health, suggest that there are three main differences between self-help groups and traditional human service agencies. A common problem or predicament is shared by all or most of the group members; there is a reciprocity of helping amongst these members and the group is self-managing. These criteria certainly apply to the SIA; all full members must be spinal cord injured, though associate members are also permitted; members help each other through the sharing of information and advice and the SIA is run by its management committee which is comprised solely of spinally injured people, although up to four others may be co-opted.

THE DEVELOPMENT OF SIA

SIA was established in 1974 in one small office with a paid general secretary and 300 members. Since then it has expanded rapidly, moved twice to larger premises and currently employs eight fulltime and four part-time staff as well as making use of a considerable number of volunteers. Membership has risen dramatically and there are now 3500 full members and 1500 associate members. The aims of the SIA, as stated in its constitution, are threefold:

1. To help individuals achieve their own goals.
2. To bring about the best medical care and rehabilitation.
3. To stimulate scientific research into paraplegia.

Before discussing how SIA attempts to meet these aims, a brief consideration of the philosophy of the organization is perhaps necessary. This philosophy encompasses both the individual and collective self-help responses discussed earlier. *Individual* members are encouraged to solve their problems themselves and not have them solved for them, though information, advice and support will be offered either from the paid staff or from other members. *Collectively* SIA aims to identify the needs of the membership as a whole and articulate these needs to statutory agencies and political parties at local and national level. Finally, it should be stressed that SIA's philosophy is not antiprofessional but concerned to co-operate and laise with professionals in order to provide a better life for all those with spinal cord injury.

The SIA management committee, run by full members, sets policies and priorities and also has a considerable input into some of the projects of the Association. The primary aim of SIA of helping members achieve their own goals is approached through two main channels – the information service and the welfare service. In addition, specialist holiday and legal services help in specific circumstances.

The information service

The information service is an essential part of the work in which all staff participate. Clearly the lack of information suggests that information is the greatest handicapping factor faced by people with disabilities. SIA seeks to spread information both through response to individual queries and through its quarterly newsletter. A conscious effort is made to distinguish the newsletter from other publications of its sort in the disability field – it is full of articles by members and of the latest ideas in the field, but contains no pictures of charities handing cheques to grateful paraplegics, or poems about coping cheerfully.

The lack of general information available to lay people about spinal cord injury led to the SIA publishing its first book, *So You're Paralysed*.[6] This was written in collaboration with a panel of experts – some doctors, some nurses, some consumers. A book on work opportunities followed,[7] then an ambitious series entitled *People with Spinal Cord Injuries: Treatment and Care*.[8] This series is aimed not at lay people but at professionals, as a response to the dearth of easily assimilated information on the subject for non-specialist professionals.

The successful growth of the SIA through the 1970s led to a realization that more than information was needed to achieve its aims: in 1980 it was decided to set up a specialist welfare service too. This was an ambitious self-help activity, as the SIA had to develop an appropriate model on which to base its welfare activities in the absence of a satisfactory existing one.

The welfare service

When looking at the provision of services for people with disabilities it would be true to say that the picture is not an inspiring one. There have been no published descriptions, let alone evaluations of service provision within disability organizations, although a number of such organizations do provide such services of one kind or another. These services were organized on a casework basis with workers either spending most of their time travelling or the service being organized on a regional basis.

A number of factors made the organization of a casework service impractical. SIA membership is spread throughout Britain and with only one worker employed it would have been an impossible task. In addition, the philosophy of the organization is a self-help one, and it was not felt that a professional casework service would make best use of the expertise within the membership. Finally, such services tend to individualize the problems of disabled people – something which the SIA is opposed to. The SIA believes that the problems of members stem from the failures and shortcomings of society rather than individual limitations.

Where professionals have concerned themselves with the problems of disability, their interventions have been based on the individual model of disability which views disability as a personal tragedy or individual disaster.[9] This approach is inappropriate; the problems of our membership were social rather than personal. Poor housing, poverty and unemployment, and lack of information, rather than the need for skilled help with coming to terms with their disabilities, were the kinds of problems which confronted our members. Consequently it was necessary to provide a service which would be appropriate to social rather than personal needs, to external rather than internal problems. That is not to deny that some members might need an individual casework service and skilled counselling help, but it was not thought appropriate to establish a welfare service which had these as prime objectives.

The idea of using community work or community social work methods as the basis for the organization of the SIA welfare service seemed attractive. The Barclay Report definition of community social work accurately describes the ethos of our service.

> By this we mean formal social work which, starting from problems affecting an individual or group and the responsibilities and resources of social services departments and voluntary organisations, seeks to tap into, support, enable and underpin the local networks of formal and informal relationships which constitute our basic definition of community, and also the strengths of a client's communities of interest. It implies, we suggest, a change of attitude on the part of social workers and their employing agencies.[10]

It is also worth pointing out that it was felt that community social work methods were appropriate to the organization of the welfare service in that SIA membership had the characteristics of what Inkeles[11] had called a 'psychic community' and what Abrams[12] had redefined as a 'moral community'. The Barclay Report had introduced another similar term, 'community of interest', but the underlying principle behind all these terms remained.

An evaluation of the work of the SIA welfare service[13] indicated the appropriateness of the model and the assumptions on which it was based. Firstly, the evaluation found that, with the exception of the medical categories, the problems experienced by members were essentially practical ones and involved with the external world: members often experience economic or housing difficulties. The second point to note is that some of the problems often assumed to figure very large in the lives of disabled people provoked few queries, especially sex, psychological problems and, perhaps surprisingly, access. One final point to note is that incontinence, while mentioned frequently, was not specifically about the inability to control one's bladder or bowels. The overwhelming queries concerned faults or problems in the equipment supplied to manage incontinence and the way suppliers – DHSS, NHS and commercial companies – often changed their products without consultation with the consumer.

There are a number of other services which are available to members or are currently being developed and these will be discussed below.

The Link scheme

The Link scheme was one of SIA's earliest services, set in action soon after the Association was formally constituted. The way it works was and is extremely simple. Members of the Association who feel they may be able to help other members, simply from their own experience, offer themselves as members of the scheme. Brief details of these people are kept on file and when the SIA office receives a request for help which in the judgement of the staff could be answered in whole or in part by contact with a Link scheme member, a suitable member of the scheme is approached and asked to contact the family or individual asking for help. The criteria used in selecting a suitable member have never been made explicit but they usually include a geographic proximity to the user of the scheme, and a similar level of lesion or other similar experience. For example, a wife of a tetraplegic will be put in touch with another wife of a tetraplegic, a young paraplegic will be put in touch with another young paraplegic and so on.

The greatest difficulty in running the scheme is the lack of personal contact between the welfare office and the Link scheme members. There is no doubt about the goodwill to be tapped within the scheme – recently a family came all the way from Birmingham to help another family in Barnet, Hertfordshire. At present the Link scheme is used no more than once or twice each week; over 200 people are registered on the scheme now, so it is unlikely that any member will be approached more than once or twice a year, although in practice some people are used more often and some are never approached. There is no way of screening or vetting Link members, but simply an informal dropping of those who are felt to be unsuitable helpers.

There is no doubt that, despite these difficulties, the Link scheme is a crucial part of the SIA welfare service overall. Not only does it provide valuable assistance to individuals at particular points in their lives, but it also makes use of the knowledge and expertise of the disabled members of the association. Hence the advantages of being part of a 'community of interest' can be passed on to those members who need it.

Counselling

Counselling for spinal cord injured people has been a topic within SIA almost since the Association's inception. The original approach was based on the view that the time of greatest need for counselling is immediately following injury, while the individual is still in hospital, and that the most appropriate people to carry out such counselling would be those who had gone through the experience before – in other words, full members of SIA. Accordingly, meetings were commenced in March 1975 with the staff of Stoke Mandeville Hospital, and a pilot counselling scheme was set up at the hospital. However, the scheme foundered after a few months and it emerged quite clearly that SIA needed to do more thinking about the type of scheme it was trying to introduce, and the practical difficulties of introducing a scheme to the largest spinal unit in the country. Some of SIAs local groups are currently in the process of establishing similar programmes in collaboration with other spinal units.

In 1978 SIA organized a counselling conference. The transcript of the conference shows consensus in three important topics. The first is the need for counselling; this was generally acknowledged, and has now been expanded to include the counselling needs of families with a disabled member, and of people who had left hospital and perhaps had been living in the community for some time. Secondly the usefulness of peer counselling was agreed; paralysed people and their families felt that they could derive greatest help from other people in a similar situation. Thirdly, and most crucially, an emphasis was placed on the need for close supervision and support for voluntary counselling.

A workshop designed to explore some of the ways in which a counselling service could be implemented within SIA was held in 1981. Nonetheless a counselling service has not been developed to any extent and, while SIA is committed to further work in this area, problems of training, supervision, control and professional suspicion remain.

The care attendant agency

The more severely disabled (tetraplegic) members of SIA had urged the management committee to look more closely at their needs, and a major survey of tetraplegic members was commissioned. The topic which emerged as of most concern for tetraplegics was carers, both the strain imposed on regular carers by lack of suitable relief, and the difficulty of getting flexible reliable help away from home. In response to this need, SIA launched its own care attendant agency, which employs three fulltime attendants, plus a number of other attendants employed on a daily rate as needed. The SIA has been fortunate in receiving excellent co-operation from the Association of Crossroads Care Attendant Schemes and Community Service Volunteers, which has offered expertise and ex-volunteers. However, the need for and existence of our agency point to the inadequacy and inflexibility of statutory-based, professionally staffed schemes like the community nursing service.

The care attendants employed by the SIA are not professionally trained, although as much informal training with members is provided as is possible. Care attendants replace the regular carer, giving personal care and doing basic household duties for members. The service is nationwide, and indeed even international. It is envisaged that in the future it could expand to help people with other disabilities.

As with all SIA services, the intention of the administration of the care attendant agency is to keep bureaucracy to a minimum. Members wishing to use the agency complete a simple booking form, and the co-ordinator selects a suitable care attendant to fit the members' needs. The usual maximum booking period is 2 weeks – this was chosen both in order to allow the SIA to spread its small resources as far as possible, and to make it clear to statutory authorities that the SIA is not seeking to replace long-term care for people with disabilities, simply to supplement services where there is an acute need for relief, or a need for care away from home.

Care attendants work in the users' own home, or travel with them as necessary. After the placement, each user is sent an evaluation form, so that the effectiveness of the service can be monitored, and a payment form. Payment is entirely voluntary, with members paying only what they can afford, or feel is reasonable, towards the service. A maximum rate of £15 per day is suggested. This is not the true cost of running the service, but is based on what was felt could reasonably be asked from SIA members, without putting off many people in need.

The service is a relatively new one, but there is no doubt that in the short time it has been running the care attendant agency has become an important part of SIAs services.

There are a number of other services that SIA offers to its members, notably a holiday service and a legal claims service. The holiday service offers special holiday facilities, including two canal boats which are specially adapted for people in wheelchairs, a mobile home in a seaside park and detailed information about suitable facilities which have been used by members in the past. The legal claims service offers the services of a qualified solicitor, himself a paraplegic, who works with members and their solicitors, helping to assess the amount of compensation to be paid following injury and the establishment of legal liability.

Several case studies, given below, provide examples of how SIAs services work.

Case study 1

A young mother became paraplegic following a road traffic accident. She was admitted to her local district general hospital. Her family contacted SIA, and asked for information about how other wheelchair-bound mothers cope. A link was arranged with a paraplegic mother in her area. SIA also sent information from the newsletter, giving personal accounts from a number of paralysed mothers. This woman subsequently went to a spinal injuries unit, and on her return to the community she contacted SIA again, for advice on choosing a car

Case study 2

A woman became paraplegic following surgery. She has considerable pain. Information on pain clinics and other therapies were sent, and a link arranged with another woman in similar circumstances. These women are still in touch with each other and SIA hears from time to time from this member as she searches for methods of pain relief.

Case study 3

A tetraplegic man contacted us for information on aids. During the conversation, problems he was having with adaptations to his kitchen and with his welfare benefits emerged. SIA gave advice on all these aspects, and wrote letters to his local authority, backing up his case on the adaptations. SIA also complained on his behalf to the local benefits office, with some success. This has developed into an ongoing relationship; he now rings SIA on a semi-regular basis, often to complain about his social services, sometimes to complain because his benefits have not been paid. As well as the practical advice and support he is given, SIA also provides a social contact.

Case study 4

A man who was contemplating marriage contacted SIA, to ask what his housing rights were, and to ask what possibility there was of him becoming a father. The association sent him information on both topics, including an article from the newsletter on male fertility. At SIA we were all very happy when a few months later he wrote to inform us that his wife was pregnant, and shortly after that wrote again announcing the birth of the baby. His case is now used to encourage other tetraplegics who may want to embark on marriage or parenthood.

SOME WAYS FORWARD

Earlier the development of SIA as a self-help group was located in its appropriate historical context. Wider economic forces have also been shaping the provision of health care generally and these also need to be considered.

Since 1953 there has been a considerable growth in social welfare expenditure both absolutely and as a proportion of gross national product. Spending on health between 1953–77 increased on average by 4.6% per year; in the same period spending on the personal social services increased by 7.6% per year and spending on social security increased by 5.1% per year. Unfortunately it is not possible to establish how much of that amount was spent specifically on disabled people but it is not unreasonable to conclude that there was a substantial improvement in the services available to disabled people. New medical technologies and treatments were developed, community health services expanded, the Chronically Sick and Disabled Persons Act established a number of new rights and services, and financial benefits like the attendance allowance, invalidity pension and mobility allowance were introduced.

However, since 1977 this rosy picture has changed and it must be noted that services to disabled people (among others) have been cut back considerably and the seriousness of the position is compounded by the fact that such services started from a very low base. At present, Britain spends considerably less on services for disabled people than almost all of its European Community neighbours. Most serious of all, the subjective experience of disability for many disabled people, and those who care for them, has improved very little despite the increased allocation of resources.

The crucial question for the 1980s is how to improve the quality of life for all of those affected by disability, during a period when it is no longer likely that there will be dramatic medical advances, or substantial extensions of existing services as a result of increased public expenditure. There are two possible answers to this question. The first involves further movement away from the delivery of health and personal services through a professionalized bureaucracy. As David Owen, one-time Minister of Health commented:

'Health is not just something that is provided for by the NHS, but that each individual has a responsibility for his own well being'.[14]

The individual can handle this responsibility in one of two ways: he/she can teach him/herself what he/she needs to know or he/she can pool his/her knowledge with that of others by joining a group. Hence the importance of SIA and other self-help groups concerned with health care.

Specifically with regard to disability, once a medical condition has been stabilized, there is no reason why the disabled person should not take responsibility for his or her own health just as everyone else does. Indeed a number of disability organizations are concerned in this area of self-help and health, as has already been discussed. Further, disabled people and their organizations are not restricting their activities to health, but also include the social consequences of disability, banding together in order to gain access to a much needed support services. Again, the emphasis of the SIA is on helping members with the emotional and practical consequences of spinal cord injury.

Often the response of the professional, when confronted with a patient or client who asserts the right to control his or her own body or social circumstances, is to doubt his or her capacity to cope and also to feel vaguely threatened by such self-assertiveness. However, there are two positive aspects to such situations. Many disabled people are more aware than anyone else of their physical conditions and the social consequences of them, simply as a result of experiencing them every single day of their lives. Further, the taking of responsibility by patients or clients removes or at least decreases the burden of responsibility upon the professional. So the SIA is concerned to show how a service based on this sharing of responsibility can actually work in practice.

It is clear that the relationship between professional and client needs to change and Finkelstein,[15] himself spinal cord injured, points to some of the directions of this change.

The basis of professional practice must rest on an assumption of integration and a commitment to promoting control by disabled people over their own lives. Since the lives of disabled people also depend on the actions of helpers, control over education, training and role of such helpers need to be vested in disabled people (quite aside from the need for more disabled people to enter the profession).

What this means in practice is that the role of the professional worker in rehabilitation, for example, needs to change from management of the patient to that of being a resource for the patient to use in reaching his or her own goals. The suggestion that professional workers in rehabilitation should become a resource to be utilized by disabled people is not a suggestion that professionals should become passive and all the onus for innovation, assessment, decision-making etc. should fall on the shoulders of disabled people. Professionals acting as a resource to be used by others need special education and training so that they are able to *promote* control by disabled people.

This accurately captures the ethos of the SIA approach – the paraplegic or tetraplegic is the expert definer of his or her own problems and needs, and the appropriate person to be in control of the rehabilitation process.

Of course it is easy for a small, flexible voluntary organization with few statutory responsibilities to develop any models of practice as and how it wishes. However, this situation does not apply to trained and qualified professionals, so the argument goes, and there are two compelling reasons for this. To begin with, most professional training is based upon the individual or medical model of disability, which it has already been suggested is inappropriate. Further, this kind of training gives a particular and false view of disability, as Scott argues:[16]

> The professional has been specially trained to give professional help to impaired people. He cannot use his expertise if those who are sent to him for assistance do not regard themselves as being impaired. Given this fact, it is not surprising that the doctrine has emerged among experts that truly effective rehabilitation and adjustment can occur only after the client has squarely faced and accepted the 'fact' that he is, indeed, 'impaired'.

For these reasons the SIA works with professionals, aiming to help them to move away from in-built conceptions of the nature of disability. It does this by providing help and advice to individual professionals, regular liaison with a variety of professional groups and making contributions to the training of various professionals, when invited.

In addition most professionals currently work in large-scale bureaucracies, with all the attendant problems of communication and co-ordination. However, the real problem is not co-ordination but, as Wilding[17] says, the consequences of services which have been built up around professional skills rather than client need.

> Services organized around professional skills are a tribute to the power of professionals in policy making. They also bear witness to a failure of professional responsibility. This is a failure to recognize that services organized around particular skills may be logical for professionals but may not meet the needs of clients and potential clients. *The real sufferers, for example, from the multiplicity of professionals actually or potentially involved in the care and rehabilitation of the physically handicapped are the handicapped.*[17] [authors' emphasis]

Finkelstein[15] suggests that the problem is not of co-ordination but of the need for a change in professional role – the professional must change from expert definer of need and/or rationer of services and become a resource which the disabled person may use as he or she chooses:

> The endemic squabbles between rehabilitation workers about professional bound-

aries and the familiar farce of professional 'teamwork' can only be put at an end when all the workers and facilities in rehabilitation become resources in a process of self-controlled rehabilitation.[15]

It is this process of 'self-controlled rehabilitation' that the SIA is seeking to promote in its contact with other professionals, particularly with spinal injuries units. Working with other disciplines from spinal units, it is clear that an individual's experience of the rehabilitation process can be far removed from the professionals' intention. It has been suggested else-where[18] that simple things, like changing the usual hospital routine, so that the patient rather than the nurse decides the time of her 2- or 3-hourly turns can help to change the medical control of disability to a rehabilitation model. It is clear that this needs a negotiated agreement between professional and patient, and probably between different disciplines of professional. As re-habilitation continues, it means allowing the individual control, allowing for decisions being changed and accepting that a tidy solution is not always the aim.

One of the SIA contentions is that a whole area of responsibility has to be given up – the professional helper has to be ready to allow disabled people to choose goals with which they do not agree. SIA also seeks to promote a spirit of generosity about the sharing of information; knowledge is often power, and this power is frequently kept in a very few hands. However, when SIA undertook a survey of its more severely disabled (tetraplegic) members, it was clear that they have an informed attitude to rehabilitation and strong opinions to contribute. Their ideas on the kind of services they would like to see for spinal injured people could apply to many sorts of disability. Two of these tetraplegic people took part in a meeting with social workers from spinal injuries units, discussing their experience of disability. Although their experiences were not unusual or even new, those professionals present re-ported learning a great deal. Just for once the consumer was the expert. By being ready to learn from consumers, the social workers in the spinal units have taken a step towards making themselves a resource rather than gate-keeper of resources. By making the consumer voice a dominant one, they have experimented with a pattern where the consumer's voice can be heard.

Voluntary organization can be the bridge of the facilitator, making the contact between consumer and worker, breaking the barriers of expectation, as well as providing a different model for services. The expectation inherent in the well/sick, doctor/patient, helper/helped way of categorizing people is that the well or the doctor or the helper *will be able* to do something for the sick, the patient, the helped. The strains imposed on the professional in try-ing to meet these expectations are only matched by the restrictions placed upon the consumer by the constructs of professional help.

The principle of self-control, which forms the cornerstone of SIAs approach to the problems of overcoming disability, is an approach which is becoming more and more relevant to professionals, both in order to resolve some of the contradictions and dissatisfactions with their own professional practice, and in order to provide a more relevant and effective service to disabled people.

REFERENCES

1. Oliver M. (1981), Disability, adjustment and family life: some theoretical considerations, in: *Handicap in a Social World* (Brechin A., Liddiard P., Swain J., eds.), Kent, Hodder & Stoughton.
2. Trieschmann R. (1980), *Spinal Cord Injuries*, Oxford, Pergamon Press.
3. Smiles S. (1866), *Self-help: with Illustrations of Character Conduct and Perseverance*, London, Murray.
4. Gosden P. (1973), *Self Help*, London, Batsford.
5. Robinson D., Henry S. (1977), *Self-Help and Health*, London, Martin Robertson.
6. Fallon B. (1975), *So You're Paralysed*, London, SIA.
7. Fallon B. (1979), *Able to Work*, London, SIA.
8. Spinal Injuries Association (1981), *People with Spinal Cord Injuries: Treatment and Care*, London, SIA.
9. Oliver M. (1983), *Social Work with Disabled People*, London, Macmillan.
10. Barclay Committee (1982), *Social Workers, their Role and Tasks*, London, Bedford Square Press.
11. Inkeles, A. (1964), *What is Sociology?* (Prentice Hall, New Jersey)
12. Abrams P. (1976), Community care: some research problems and priorities, in: *Social Care Research* (Barnes J., Connelly, N., eds.), London, Bedford Square Press.
13. Oliver M., Hasler F. (1983), *Social Work in a Self-help Group*, London, SIA.
14. Owen D. (1976), *The Times*.
15. Finkelstein V. (1981), *Disability and Professional Attitudes*, Sevenoaks, NAIDEX Conventions.
16. Scott R. A. (1970), Deviance and respectability in Douglas J. D. (ed.) *Construction of Conceptions of Stigma by Professional Experts*, New York, Basic Books.
17. Wilding P. (1982), *Professional Power and Social Welfare*, London, Routledge & Kegan Paul.
18. Hasler F., Anderson A. (1984), Rhetoric or reality. *Community Care*, 6.9.1984.

13

Services provided by the local authority

Michael Brill

INTRODUCTION

A time will come in the course of most disabling diseases when the intervention of the medical and rehabilitative services will show decreasing returns. The person ceases to be a patient, moves out of the medical umbrella, and has to start living a life as normally as possible, albeit at a reduced level of functioning. It is at this point, in the United Kingdom, when both the local authority and agencies other than the health services of central government, start to have a role to play.

At this time of change in the career of disabled people two major problems confront them. Firstly, they face the problems caused by loss of income-earning capacity and by the fact that their disability forces them into extra expenditure for transport etc. Secondly, they need help in the non-financial consequences of their disability. In the United Kingdom the responsibility for maintaining their income at a certain minimum level falls on the social security system of central government. The alleviation of the non-financial consequences of disability is largely the responsibility of the local authority.

Like hospitals and health authorities, some local authorities are good, some are indifferent and some provide an unsatisfactory service. However, unlike the health services the local authority is subject to local elected control. The consequence of this is that the range, quantity and quality of service will vary considerably from one authority to another. A paper such as this can only give an overview of the range of services that may be provided. It is highly unlikely that all the services will be available in any one area. That being said, all local authorities have certain specific duties to help disabled people, irrespective of their degree of disability. It is their task to provide the caring services that do not need the skills of a trained nurse and pressure can be brought to bear to get them to provide the services needed.

Within the local authority several different departments will have some responsibilities towards disabled people. For example, the finance department will be involved with the rating relief of property specially adapted for disabled people; the planning department is involved in ensuring access by wheelchair users to public places; the education department will be involved in the provision of special education for disabled children and special classes such as lip-reading classes for adults; the local swimming baths may well run special classes for disabled people and the library service will be providing large-print books for the partially sighted and perhaps a house-bound readers' service.

However, one department above all others has responsibility to provide services for disabled people. The social services departments were set up in 1971 to provide a wide range of welfare services to people with difficulties and handicaps. A social services department will be headed by a director of social services who is answerable to a committee of elected members. The normal first point of contact for disabled people and their helpers will be an area or divisional team or the social services department in a hospital; the staff of this team will be employed by the local authority and not by the hospital. There is no need for a medical referral and indeed most departments would prefer the approach to come from handicapped people themselves. From this point of contact the disabled person should have access to services ranging from full residential care through the provision of domiciliary services such as home helps, to something as simple as the provision of a bath seat to help getting in and out of the bath. In addition, area and hospital social work teams should be able to provide a source of advice and expertise about other resources and services for disabled people in the local area. General support should also be given to assist with coping with the emotional consequences of handicap.

HOUSING AND ACCOMMODATION

A fundamental need for everyone is for accommodation, but for disabled people the problems can be particularly pressing. Most newly disabled people return to their own homes where severe problems may arise from the unsuitability of their accommodation for disabled living. For others, particularly if they are homeless and rootless, their previous lifestyle is impossible given their handicap. For a final group, the severity of their handicap leads to an assumption that they would not be able to live outside institutional care. For all these people a responsibility rests on the local authority to ensure that they are adequately accommodated.

To deal first with those people returning to their own home, the local authority has a responsibility to ensure that the disabled person is able to live there. This can lead to a need for extensive alterations. Doors need to be made wide enough for wheelchair access; kitchens must be adapted to the needs of the handicapped cook; lavatories, baths and showers need to be altered or installed to suit the person's changed circumstances. This can be accomplished in a variety of ways, depending on the nature of the property and whether it is owned or rented by the disabled person. In some circumstances the changes can be made by the preferential award of improvement grants available to improve the general quality of housing; sometimes by direct grants from the social services department to alleviate specific problems caused by the disability; and sometimes, where the disabled person is already living in council-owned accommodation, by using the authority's general housing powers to improve its own accommodation. In addition, where part of the home has been adapted specifically to the needs of the handicapped person, that part becomes eligible for rating relief.

The amount of help that will be given however will vary substantially from person to person and from authority to authority. It makes sense to install an expensive stairlift or build an outside bathroom for a young disabled person with many years to live. An elderly person or someone who is likely to die in the near future is more likely to be offered cheaper, less satisfactory help. This may be as cheap and as crude as the offer of the loan of a chemical toilet to obviate the need to climb the stairs to the bathroom (see p. 23). The amount and nature of the help are largely discretionary and vary from one authority to another. The level of adaptation offered may even critically depend on the judgement of the person from the local authority who makes the assessment of need.

The problem is somewhat greater when the disabled person has no adaptable property to return to. This can happen for a number of reasons. Some people have no real base and these are often people whose previous lifestyle led them into particular danger of injury. For others, their previous accommodation may be totally unsuitable for adaptation. For a third, particularly sad group, one of the consequences of their disability will be that their marriages or other living arrangements are broken up.

Where a disabled person becomes homeless for such a reason, then the housing authority has specific responsibilities to rehouse him or her as a homeless vulnerable person. Most housing authorities have a small stock of more or less well adapted accommodation and all have the power to alter and adapt existing premises to suit the person's specific needs. In other cases warden-assisted accommodation may be available either as part of a complex largely meant for elderly people or, much more rarely, in a block solely designed for younger disabled people.

However, the housing department's resources are not solely confined to property owned by the council. In particular the housing department often works closely with local housing associations to provide specialist accommodation. Access to housing association accommodation is usually via application to the association, but sometimes housing departments have direct nomination rights.

Housing departments can also be good or bad and there is enormous local variation. The problem is compounded by the fact that in many parts of the country, the housing authority is a different tier of local government from the social services department and this can lead to major problems of co-operation and co-ordination. Housing is scarce in most parts of the country and waiting lists are long. However whereas able-bodied people can be housed in temporary accommodation, disabled people cannot so easily be catered for. In such circumstances it is tempting for the housing association to leave a disabled person in a hospital or a home or to suggest that the person is far too handicapped ever to live independently.

Residential care

Housing departments and others are, to a certain extent, encouraged to support residential care because of a commonly held but fallacious view that many people are so disabled that they are destined to spend the rest of their lives in some sort of institution. The facts do not bear this out. Whilst there remain many mentally handicapped, mentally ill or elderly people, who are likely to spend their life in institutional care, this is not the case where a person under 65 is suffering from a purely physical disability. There is currently some provision for them, provided both by health authorities and by social services authorities, but this is limited. In one local authority and coterminous health authority area with a population of 156 000, 1940 people under the age of 65 were registered with the local authority as handicapped. Of these, only 41 were in residential care. Of these, 11 were in hospital beds, including 4 in the local psychiatric hospital. Nearly all the 41 suffered either from a coexisting psychiatric disorder or had damaged institutionalized personalities. Four were suffering from the terminal stages of degenerative neurological conditions. Theoretically, health authorities should be making provision for handicapped people where there is a need for a high input of skilled nursing care that could not be provided by the district nursing service, whilst the local authority should be providing for those people who do not need such skilled care, but in practice the division is not so clear-cut. Chance and the availability of places are more likely to be the determining factors.

Health authorities have in the past been expected to make provision for handicapped people in younger disabled units and a level of provision of between 6 and 20 per 100 000 population has been suggested, but these guidelines have been honoured more in the breach than in the observance. There are no useful equivalent guidelines for the provision of non-hospital residential care and this is even more a matter for local determination. Provision can range from that which is excellent to that which is frankly terrible. Some accommodation is in small home-like residences where disabled people have their own bedrooms, staff levels are high, and the whole establishment is geared around philosophies which give back to disabled people control of their own lives. Too often, however, the accommodation is in gaunt relics of the Victorian era, in colonies designed to keep disabled people out of sight and where the 20-bedded dormitory is the norm. Some social services departments own and run their own accommodation, but more frequently they will sponsor placement in establishments run by the voluntary sector. A good example of this sort of provision is that provided by the Leonard Cheshire Foundation (see Chapter 14).

In recent years social service departments have been withdrawing to a considerable extent from the provision of residential care at all. This is the result of a change in funding arrangements whereby the social security system funds residential placements, leaving the local authority only with the responsibility of topping up the funding of very expensive placements.

When all is said and done, the provision of residential care is a blind alley. It affects only a tiny proportion of all disabled people and it is expensive. Most of all it tends to add to the handicap of disabled people by putting them in unnatural living situations which help to mark them out and separate them from the world at large. One of the major worries is that often it is a speciously simple solution to a difficult problem, but one which takes no account of the civil rights of disabled people. Like every one else except prisoners and those detained in psychiatric hospital, physically handicapped people have an absolute right to live in the community. Unlike others however, they often depend on others to help them achieve this.

HELP IN THE COMMUNITY

What physically disabled people need is not institutional care but a replacement for the limbs and organs they lack or which do not function well. It is a primary task of the social services department to compensate for this lack and to help the disabled person lead as full a life as possible. Once the matter of accommodation is settled then there are two ways that help can be given. The first approach must be to work to make the person as independent as possible without the intervention of other people. This largely means the provision of mechanical aids which facilitate the performance of the functions of daily living. Like so much in this area, there is considerable overlap between those devices provided by the local authority and those provided by the health authority. Moreover the central government agencies have specific responsibilities to provide certain very expensive resources and certain aids specifically designed to help the disabled person function at work. In the main it is the responsibility of the health authority to provide those aids which help the nursing function, and the social services department has the responsibility for providing aids which help in the normal process of daily living. Many such aids are very simple. Adapted cutlery is a good example. The provision of a Nelson knife may mean that a disabled person is not dependent on someone else for cutting up food. Aids can be much more complex however. Mechanical hoists with tracking can minimize the dependence of a severely disabled person on others for mobility, and the provision of a stairlift can open up the top part of the house again. The difficulty arises in deciding what aids are needed as a direct result of disablement and what is equipment which is needed for daily living but is only marginally related to the disablement. A disabled housewife may be able to function better with a top-loading washing machine rather than the front-loader she already owns. It would however be unusual for this to be provided by a social services department. This problem is likely to be compounded by the surfeit of devices produced as a spin-off of the computer revolution, providing new and exciting solutions to the problems of communication and environmental control. For example, one interesting area of development which is becoming widely available is the provision of call alarm systems allowing handicapped people to live alone (see p. 186).

Mechanical devices can only provide limited solutions however and the fundamental need for many disabled people is for the help of other human beings to carry out the activities needed to compensate for the handicaps caused by the disability. For this essential service disabled people mainly depend on the unsung and unpaid services of their relatives and friends. In comparison with the help given by these people, that given by the statutory services is relatively unimportant. Moreover without this largely unpaid help the statutory services are unlikely to be able to cope with the press of need. Consequently, one of the tasks of the social services departments is to support and sustain the informal care network. This is a task which on the whole is badly completed. Caring relatives are left with far too high a burden of care, because they do not complain. Alternatively the pattern of relief care offered is governed by what is on offer, rather than what is needed. There is however much that could be done to help relatives and friends, ranging from the provision of relief care when the responsibility is taken over for greater or less periods of time, to the support and sustaining of the voluntary groups and relatives' groups which are set up to help.

It is a fundamental part of the task of the social services department to provide staff to relieve relatives and friends or to provide help when none other is available. This has been a service traditionally and effectively carried out by the district nursing service, but increasingly other methods of relieving the nursing service are being explored to enable them to carry out specific nursing functions. The home help service is the best established of the alternative caring services, largely caring for elderly people, but also able to provide a useful service to younger disabled people. Traditionally the home help was provided to undertake domestic tasks such as cooking, cleaning and shopping. Following adoption of a new nationally agreed job description home helps can now be expected to be involved with intimate personal tasks such as washing, dressing or toilet duties. However it is inevitable and admirable that many home helps become increasingly involved in tasks well outside their formal job descriptions. To a great extent the home care service still has its roots in the traditions of voluntarism and home helps are often reported to spend significant periods of time helping disabled people outside the specific periods for which they are paid.

The other long-standing social service which needs to be identified here is the meals on wheels service. Sometimes organized and run by voluntary organizations such as the Women's Royal Voluntary Service and sometimes run directly by the authority itself, it is a very well known service but perhaps not as efficient as would appear at first sight.

Both the meals on wheels service and the home care service were set up in the immediate post-war period as a response to conditions that existed at that time. The home care service, for example, was originally set up as a response to needs of new mothers in the days immediately following the birth of their baby. Over time these services have grown and changed in response to changing circumstances. They are perhaps now at a point where they are likely to go through a period of radical reappraisal. The primary tasks that now need to be undertaken are those which can reasonably be expected of a competent caring relative, rather than those carried out by a domestic or cleaner. The implications of this are that the years to come will see the inevitable raising of the status and pay of home care workers with a concomitant widening of the range of tasks that they are able to undertake.

Some tentative first steps have been taken in the development in some areas of care attendant schemes (see also pp. 191–3, 242). Like many of the best ideas this has largely been developed and sustained in the voluntary sector and is usually known as a crossroads scheme, after a character in a well known soap opera, and there are powerful arguments for leaving the initiative with the voluntary sector. Details are available from the Association of Crossroads Care Attendant Schemes (Chapter 14). Problems do arise about the funding of such a relatively expensive service and in some areas no voluntary organization comes forward to run it. Consequently in some areas experiments in which the local authority provides the care attendants are being tried, sometimes as a joint venture with the health authority.

Another exciting area of development has been the expanding use of young volunteers who come for periods of between 4 and 6 months to be the arms and legs of disabled people. For this they are given only their board, lodging and pocket money and are usually supported and supervised by the local social services department.

Finally, a more traditional method which often provides vital relief for handicapped person and helper alike is the provision of cheap or free holidays for the handicapped person. This can provide a break for the carer, and at the same time is an enjoyable experience for the handicapped person (p. 188).

DAY CARE

Another response to the problem of providing care for disabled people is the provision of day centres for physically handicapped people. Day centres have very different historical origins to those of the domiciliary services, stemming as they do from attempts to provide gainful employment for the badly damaged men returning from the trenches of World War I. In a limited number of places sheltered workshops exist, run in conjunction with central government, and there are also residual schemes for the blind, usually run and organized by local associations and for which the local authority is empowered to maintain minimum wage rates no matter how much or little the blind person produces.

However the real flowering of day centres for the physically handicapped came in the 1970s during a major expansion of the social services. Some carried on the tradition of providing work, taking in subcontracted light assembly and packing work from local factories. Major problems arise in such situations about rates of pay because earnings need to be drastically limited if the disabled person is not to lose social security entitlement. The provision of ill paid unskilled routine work also makes less sense in a time of high unemployment when there is little chance of a day centre providing a stepping stone to outside employment.

Day centres have therefore been providing a wide range of services which are empirically seen to be useful without necessarily having a clear and explicit task or function. One purpose is of course the provision of substitute care whilst the normal carers are doing other things. Another primary task is the provision of primary care services such as bathing where the home has been ill adapted for the task or to relieve the nursing service. Many day centres are however ill equipped to carry out these tasks, having been set up in unadapted property without proper baths or toilets etc. Moreover both these functions imply high staffing levels and the provision of much personal care. Many local authorities would not see this as a function of day centres.

There is a higher level of agreement about the provision of diversional activities in day centres. Such day provision works on the principle that disabled people are more likely to become unhappy and depressed because of their lack of functioning than the able-bodied. They therefore need to be given opportunities to undertake stimulating and worthwhile activities to give them some purpose in life. This is an aim that is often not fulfilled. In the less inspired day centres, disabled people can be left doing unimaginative craftwork. Other centres are more planned and structured in their organization of activities and, rather than providing craftwork as an end in itself, are exploring ways of enabling disabled people to lead fulfilled and successful lives in a world in which they are unlikely to be offered paid employment ever again. Such approaches depend on the disabled people recognizing that they still have many skills and abilities which they can offer to others. Thus the ex-accountant can take over the treasurership of a local organization or the handicapped housewife can help with local literacy schemes.

Such approaches differ from more traditional ones in attempting to move away from situations where the able-bodied helper does things for and to disabled people, to one where disabled people are in a more equal partnership with able-bodied people (see also pp. 127–9).

ACCESS

The provision of day care highlights some of the central dilemmas in the provision of services for disabled people. They do have specific special needs and problems which are not shared with the able-bodied and often it is easier to recognize the needs and common problems that they share with other disabled people rather than the needs and problems they share with the able-bodied. This is not necessarily what disabled people want. The provision of transport provides a good case study. For many disabled people the problem of getting around outside is the major handicap. Local authority strategies to provide help have been two-pronged. One strategy is to help in the provision of mass transport. Most local authorities run fleets of vehicles, often with tail lifts to take disabled people to and from day care. They are often also used to take people to and from social clubs, classes and to other activities specifically designed for them. Running ambulance fleets in this way is a high-profile activity. As the ambulances go around the authority in the council livery they are a concrete and well accepted demonstration of rates expenditure. They are however a very high-cost resource, often being staffed with both driver and escort whether disabled people need this level of supervision or not. Moreover they can only go to a limited number of places and so disabled people are inevitably brought together with other disabled people, rather than being given the opportunity of spending their time with non-disabled people.

In a certain very limited number of authorities more adventurous methods of improving the mobility of disabled people are being tried. Ordinary public transport is being made accessible to wheelchair users. Taxi services running specially adapted vehicles are being subsidized by local authorities and local voluntary organizations are supported in running and co-ordinating existing transport in a more flexible way.

The other way for the local authority to help is by increasing the individual's mobility in two ways. Local authorities are responsible for administering disabled drivers (and passengers) schemes, whereby privileged parking arrangements can be made available for those suffering from severe mobility problems. This can however be a benefit of limited value unless it is part of a wider strategy of providing access (see also pp. 139–42).

At one level the planning departments and other departments with inspectorial functions, such as the fire brigade, are those having the most fundamental effect on the lives of disabled people. On the one hand they can, with imagination, be a benign force by implementing a comprehensive policy. Local authorities do have powers to insist that public buildings are made accessible to disabled people, but too often even something as fundamental as local authority polling stations cannot be reached by people in wheelchairs. Providing access is an expensive business. Too often planning and inspection powers are used in an unconstructive way. For example, wheelchair users are denied admission to theatres on specious safety and fire risk grounds. Sometimes planning controls are used to support and give strength to community prejudice about disabled people.

EDUCATION

The integration of disabled people into the community at large cannot only be dealt with by the provision of technical access devices. Education departments have as great or a greater part to play.

Traditionally, disabled children have been educated separately. It was felt that they needed small classes and special teaching to help with their particular problems. This inevitably led to separate education, often in boarding schools where the care and nurture after school hours was less than good. Moreover the provision of separate residential schooling could in some cases strain the links with parents and families who were already having difficulties in accepting damaged children. The result could be emotional harm to add to the already existing physical impairment. Even the provision of separate day education has been shown to have deleterious effects, both causing stigmatization and by preventing the children from sharing their lives with other children in the streets by sending them to different schools, often involving long and exhausting journeys.

In the field of education, concepts of integration have been carried further than in many other areas. Procedures which now need to be followed before a child is given separate special education have been made much more rigorous and in particular the medical, educational, psychological and social reports have to explain specifically and clearly why separate education is essential. These reports are made available to the parents who have a right of appeal against the decision. As a result, more and more disabled children are being educated with their peers and an inevitable consequence of this is that more non-disabled children will have direct experience of disabled children. Concepts of integration may therefore be more widely accepted in future years.

CONCLUSIONS

In the final analysis the direct intervention of the local authority should only be a peripheral factor in the provision of support for disabled people. Local authorities cannot cure the disability, nor is it their job. The direct task they do have is to compensate in various ways for people's disability, largely by the provision of direct service. There are however two major disadvantages that stem from the fact that it is the local authority which provides the service. Firstly, it is paternalistic and inevitably takes control from the disabled person. For example, if the local authority provides a home help then it is the local authority rather than the disabled person who decides the level of cleanliness of the home. If the disabled person is in residential care the paternalism can be even more intrusive, even laying down rules about such personal activities as the person's sex life. Secondly, the provision of service can often be more efficiently and cheaply provided on a mass basis. Disabled people are brought together without consideration given to whether this is what they want. Disabled people are not a class identified by common desires. They are a group identified only by common handicaps and disabilities.

Better solutions rest in the areas of income maintenance devices. Perhaps the most common handicap disabled people face is a loss of usable income, both by the diminution of earning power and because disablement leads to significant added expense. Income maintenance is however not the task of the local authority but rests instead with central government. Perhaps it will be necessary to await a more favourable economic climate before significant improvement can be made to the daily lot of disabled people.

14

Some useful names and addresses

Throughout this book the different ways in which the voluntary sector may be of help to disabled individuals has been emphasized. Usually these references have been to charities concerned with helping people suffering from a particular illness or particular kind of disability. Often such bodies are able to give advice to their members on the many problems they are likely to experience personally, financially, at work and within society at large. Many people, however, have not joined appropriate self-help groups, and are not aware of the different benefits, both financial and otherwise, to which they are entitled. An enormous amount of information is published annually by the Disability Alliance (see below) in the Disability Rights Handbook. This is a guide to rights, benefits and services for all people with disabilities and their families, and is an invaluable source of information. Most of the names and addresses in this chapter can be found in the Disability Rights Handbook and the useful names and addresses mentioned below are those which the authors have found helpful in the past, or which have been referred to in other parts of the book.

This list is not comprehensive. We hope, however, that it will provide useful insight for professional people into the variety of self-help groups available, together with useful addresses of government or other agencies which are also important resources.

Information about organizations not listed, or about regional organizations, may be obtained from:

Northern Ireland Council on Disability, 2 Annadale Avenue, Belfast BT7 3JR. Tel. 0232 491011

Royal Association for Disability and Rehabilitation (RADAR), 25 Mortimer Street, London W1N 8AB. Tel. 01 637 5400

Scottish Council on Disability, Princes House, 5 Shandwick Place, Edinburgh EH2 4RG. Tel. 031 229 8632

Wales Council for the Disabled, Caerbragdy Industrial Estate, Bedwas Road, Caerphilly, Mid Glamorgan CF8 3SL. Tel. 0222 887325

USEFUL ADDRESSES

Action for Research into Multiple Sclerosis (ARMS), 4a Chapel Hill, Stansted, Essex CM24 8AG. Tel. 0279 815553

Age Concern, Bernard Sunley House, 60 Pitcairn Road, Mitcham, Surrey CR4 3LL. Tel. 01 640 5431

AID Finance, 183 Brighton Road, Coulsdon, Surrey CR3 2NF. Tel. 01 645 9014

Arthritis and Rheumatism Council, 41 Eagle Street, London WC1R 4AR. Tel. 01 405 8572

Arthritis Care, 6 Grosvenor Crescent, London SW1X 7ER. Tel. 01 235 0902

Association of Carers, 21–23 New Road, Chatham, Kent ME4 4QJ. Tel. 0634 813981

Association of Continence Advisers, c/o Disabled Living Foundation (see p. 264)

Association of Crossroads Care Attendant Schemes, 10 Regent Place, Rugby, Warwickshire CV21 2PN. Tel. 0788 73653

Association of Disabled Professionals, The Stables, 73 Pound Road, Banstead, Surrey SM7 2HU. Tel. 07373 52366

Association for Spina Bifida and Hydrocephalus (ASBAH), 22 Upper Woburn Place, London WC1H 0EP. Tel. 01 388 1382

Association of Swimming Therapy, Mr. T. Cowen (Secretary), 4 Oak Street, Shrewsbury SY3 7RH. Tel. 0743 4393

Attendance Allowance Unit, DHSS, North Fylde Central Office, Norcross, Blackpool FY5 3TA. Tel. 0253 856 123

Back Pain Association, 31–33 Park Road, Teddington, Middlesex TW11 0AB. Tel. 01 977 5474

BACUP (British Association of Cancer United Patients), 121/123 Charterhouse Street, London EC1M 6AA. Tel. 01 608 1661

Banstead Place Mobility Centre, Park Road, Banstead, Surrey SM7 3EE. Tel. 07373 51674

Break (holidays for disabled), 20 Hooks Hill Road, Sheringham, Norfolk NR26 8NL. Tel. 0263 823170

Breast Care and Mastectomy Association of Great Britain, 26A Harrison Street, Off Grays Inn Road, London WC1H 8JG. Tel. 01 837 0908

British Association of Cancer United Patients–see BACUP.

British Colostomy Association, 38–39 Eccleston Square, London SW1V 1PB. Tel. 01 828 5175

British Council for Organisations of Disabled People, St Mary's Church, Greenlaw Street, Woolwich, London SE19 5AR. Tel. 01 316 4184

British Diabetic Association, 10 Queen Anne Street, London W1M 0BD. Tel. 01 323 1531

British Epilepsy Association, 92–94 Tooley Street, London SE1 9SF. Tel. 01 403 4111

British Heart Foundation, 102 Gloucester Place, London W1H 4DH. Tel. 01 935 0185

British League Against Rheumatism, 41 Eagle Street, London WC1R 4AR. Tel. 01 405 8572

British Red Cross Society, 9 Grovenor Crescent, London SW1X 7EJ. Tel. 01 235 5454

British School of Motoring, 119 The Broadway, Wimbledon, London SW19. Tel. 01 543 5554

British Sports Association for the Disabled, Hayward House, Barnard Crescent, Aylesbury HP21 9PP. Tel. 0296 27889

British Thoracic Society, 1 St Andrews Place, Regents Park, London NW1 4LB. Tel. 01 486 7766

Camping for the Disabled, 20 Burton Close, Dawley, Telford, Shropshire. TF4 2BX. Tel. (by day) 0743 77489 (by night) 0952 507653

Cancerlink, 17 Britannia Street, London WC1X 9JN. Tel. 01 833 2451

Cancer Research Campaign, 2 Carlton House Terrace, London SW1Y 5AR. Tel. 01 930 8972

Centre on the Environment for the Handicapped, 35 Great Smith Street, London SW1P 3BJ. Tel. 01 222 7980

Chest, Heart and Stroke Association, Tavistock House North, Tavistock Square, London WC1H 9JE. Tel. 01 387 3012

Colostomy Welfare Group, See British Colostomy Association (see p. 262)

Department of Transport, Disability Unit, 2 Marsham Street, London SW1P 3EB. Tel. 01 212 4431

Derby Disabled Driving Centre, Kingsway Hospital, Kingsway, Derby DE3 LZ. Tel. 0332 371929

Design and Manufacture for Disability (DEMAND), 99 Leman Street, London E1 8EY. Tel. 01 488 9869

DIAL UK, Dial House, 117 High Street, Clay Cross, Chesterfield, Derbyshire S45 9DZ. Tel. 0246 864498

Disability Alliance ERA, 25 Denmark Street, London WC2H 8NJ. Tel. 01 240 0806

Disabled Drivers Association, Ashwellthorpe Hall, Ashwellthorpe, Norfolk NR6 1EX. Tel. 050 841 449

Disabled Drivers Motor Club, Cottingham Way, Thrapston, Northants NN14 4PL.. Tel. 0801 24724

Disabled Housing Trust, Ernest Kleinwort Court, Oakenfield, Burgess Hill, West Sussex RH15 8SJ. Tel. 04446 47892

Disabled Information Service, 105 Long Street, Atherstone, Warwickshire CV9 1AB. Tel. 08277 67020

Disabled Living Foundation, 380 Harrow Road, London W9 2HU. Tel. 01 289 6111

Disabled Motorists Federation, National Mobility Centre, Unit 2a, Atcham Estate, Shrewsbury SY4 4UG. Tel. 074 377 489

Disablement Income Group, Millmead Business Centre, Millmead Road, London N17 9QU. Tel. 01 801 8013

Disablement Services Branch, 6a Government Buildings, Warbreck Hill Road, Blackpool FY2 0UZ. Tel. 0253 856123

Driver and Vehicle Licensing Centre, Swansea SA99 1AB. Tel. 0792 72151

Electronic Equipment Loan Service for Disabled People, Willowbrook, Swanbourne Road, Mursley, Milton Keynes, Buckinghamshire MK17 0JA. Tel. 029672 533

Gardens for the Disabled Trust, Little Dane, Biddenden, Kent TN27 8JT. Tel. 0580 291214

General Medical Council, 44 Hallam Street, London W1N 6AE. Tel. 01 580 7642

Head Injuries Rehabilitation Centre, 29 Exeter Road, Selly Oak, Birmingham B29 6EX. Tel. 021 472 1083

Headway, National Head Injuries Association, 200 Mansfield Road, Nottingham NG1 3HX. Tel. 0602 622382

Health Education Authority, Hamilton House, Mabledon Place, London WC1H 9TX. Tel. 01 631 0930

Help the Aged, St James Walk, London EC1R 0BE. Tel. 01 253 0253

Ileostomy Association of Great Britain, Amblehurst House, Chobham, Woking, Surrey GU24 8PZ. Tel. 0623 28099

Incontinence Advisory Service, c/o Disabled Living Foundation, 380–384 Harrow Road, London W9 2HU. Tel. 01 289 6111

Intractable Pain Society of GB and N Ireland, Dr. T. P. Nash (Hon. Secretary), Basingstoke District Hospital, Aldermaston Road, Basingstoke RG24 9NA. Tel. 0256 473202

Jubilee Sailing Trust, Test Road, Easton Dock, Southampton SO1 1UG. Tel. 0703 631 388

John Grooms Association for the Disabled, 10 Gloucester Drive, Finsbury Park, London N4 2LP. Tel. 01 802 7272

Kingston Trust, The Drove, Kempshott, Basingstoke, Hampshire RG22 5LU. Tel. 0256 52320

Leonard Cheshire Foundation, 26–29 Maunsel Street, London SW1P 2QN. Tel. 01 828 1822

Leukaemia Care Society, PO Box 82, Exeter EX2 5DP. Tel. 0392 218514

Leukaemia Research Fund, 43 Great Ormond Street, London WC1N 3JJ. Tel. 01 405 0101

Medical Disability Society, c/o Dr F. Middleton, Hon. Secretary, Royal National Orthopaedic Hospital, Stanmore HA7 4LP. Tel. 01 954 2300

Mobility Allowance Unit, DHSS, North Fylde Central Office, Norcross, Blackpool FY5 3TA. Tel. 0253 856123

Mobility Information Service, Unit 2a, Atcham Industrial Estate, Upton Magna, Shrewsbury SY4 4UG. Tel. 0743 77489

Motability, 61 Southwark Street, London SE1 08F. Tel. 01 620 0400

Motor Neurone Disease Association, 61 Derngate, Northampton NN1 1UE.

Multiple Sclerosis Society of Great Britain and Northern Ireland, 25 Effie Road, London SW6 1EE. Tel. 01 736 6267

National Ankylosing Spondylitis Society, 6 Grosvenor Crescent, London SW1X 7ER. Tel. 01 235 9585

National Association of Laryngectomy Clubs, 39 Eccleston Square, London SW1V 1PB. Tel. 01 834 2857

National Association for Mental Health, (MIND), 22 Harley Street, London W1N 2ED. Tel. 01 637 0741

National Association of Swimming Clubs for the Handicapped, c/o Mr. J. A. Burgin, Room 401, 2 Cheapside, Reading RG1 7AA. Tel. 0734 505394

National Council of Voluntary Organisations, 26 Bedford Square, London WC1B 3HU. Tel. 01 636 4066

Opportunities for the Disabled, 1 Bank Buildings, Princes Street, London EC2R 8EU. Tel. 01 726 4963

Outset, 18 Creekside, London SE8 3DZ. Tel. 01 692 7141

Parkinson's Disease Society of the UK, 36 Portland Place, London W1N 3DG. Tel. 01 323 1174

Patients Association, Room 33, 18 Charing Cross Road, London WC2H 0HR. Tel. 01 240 0671

Physically Handicapped and Able Bodied (PHAB), Tavistock House North, Tavistock Square, London WC1H 9HX. Tel. 01 388 1963

Princess Margaret Rose Orthopaedic Hospital, Fairmilehead, Edinburgh EH10 7ED. Tel. 031 445 4123

Rehabilitation Engineering Movement Advisory Panels (REMAP), 25 Mortimer Street, London W1N 8AB. Tel. 01 637 5400

Royal Hospital and Home, Putney, West Hill, London SW15 3SW. Tel. 01 788 4511

Royal Society for Mentally Handicapped Children and Adults (MENCAP), 123 Golden Lane, London EC1Y 0RT. Tel. 01 253 9433

St Loyes College for Training the Disabled for Commerce and Industry, Fairfield House, Topsham Road, Exeter, Devon EX2 6EP. Tel. 0392 55428

Scleroderma Society, Membership Secretary, 32 Wensleydale Road, Hampton, Middlesex TW12 2LW. Tel. 01 941 4135

SEQUAL (formerly Possum Users Association), Ddol Hir, Glyn Ceirlog, Llangollen, Clwyd. Tel. 0691 72 331

Sexual and Personal Relationships of the Disabled (SPOD), 286 Camden Road, London N7 0BJ. Tel. 01 607 8851/2

Spastics Society, 12 Park Crescent, London W1N 4EQ. Tel. 01 636 5020

Spinal Injuries Association, New Point House, 76 St James Lane, London N10 3DF. Tel. 01 444 2121

Talking Books for the Handicapped National Listening Library, 12 Lant St, London SE1 1QH. Tel. 01 407 9417

Trans-Care International, 193–195 High Street, Acton, London W3 9DD. Tel. 01 992 5077

Wessex Rehabilitation Association, Odstock Hospital, Salisbury, Wiltshire SP2 8BJ. Tel. 0722 336262

Winged Fellowship Trust, Angel House, Pentonville Road, London N1 9XD. Tel. 01 833 2594

Index